Making amends

In the 1980s in Europe and North America we witnessed a remarkable revival of interest in reparation ('making amends') by offenders to their victims as an alternative to the more usual forms of punishment. In England and Wales the Home Office was (briefly) infected by this enthusiasm. Experiments were run, research was commissioned, expectations were raised.

This book critically examines those experiments. The author was granted a unique insight into the practice of reparation schemes; he found that the schemes were committed to traditional probation service objectives (diversion, mitigation, and offender education), rather than to the principle that victims had a right to reparation and offenders a corresponding obligation. In part, therefore, this book examines the practice of reparation schemes; but it is also a study of the intractability of our criminal justice institutions. These experiments reflected an abiding dissatisfaction with criminal courts and with the manner in which justice is conceived and expressed within the criminal framework. In that sense the reparation initiative was important and the vision which it largely failed to realise is bound to endure.

In addition to the author's account of reparation in the UK, *Making Amends* includes comparative studies written by researchers based in Germany and the United States.

'I am of the firm opinion that this book is by far the most thoughtful, well-written and knowledgeable book to be written on this subject. Davis has used reparation and mediation to explore in a very stimulating way questions central to the principles of criminal justice and ideas such as just deserts, utilitarianism, and the boundary between criminal and civil law.'

Mike Maguire, *University of Wales, Cardiff*

Making amends

Mediation and reparation in criminal justice

Gwynn Davis

with Heinz Messmer, Mark S. Umbreit and
Robert B. Coates

ROUTLEDGE

London and New York

First published in 1992
by Routledge
2 Park Square, Milton Park, Abingdon, Oxon, OX14 4RN (UK)

Simultaneously published in the USA and Canada
by Routledge
711 Third Avenue, New York, NY 10017 (US)

First issued in paperback 2013

Routledge is an imprint of the Taylor & Francis Group, an informa business

© 1992 The volume as a whole: Gwynn Davis; Chapter 9: Heinz
Messmer; Chapter 10: Mark S. Umbreit and Robert B. Coates

Typeset by LaserScript, Mitcham, Surrey

British Library Cataloguing in Publication Data
Davis, Gwynn
Making amends: mediation and reparation in criminal justice.
I. Title II. Messmer, Heinz III. Umbreit, Mark
364.68

Library of Congress Cataloging in Publication Data
Davis, Gwynn
Making amends: mediation and reparation in criminal justice / by
Gwynn Davis with Heinz Messmer, Mark Umbreit, and Robert Coates.
p. cm.
Includes bibliographical references and index.
1. Reparation – Great Britain. 2. Victims of crimes – Legal status, laws,
etc. – Great Britain. 3. Mediation – Great Britain. 4. Criminal justice,
Administration of – Great Britain.
KD2007.D38 1992
344.41'03288 – dc20
[344.1043288]
91-37595
CIP

ISBN 0–415–06708–1
ISBN 978-0-415-86213-4 (Paperback)

Publisher's Note

The publisher has gone to great lengths to ensure the quality of this reprint
but points out that some imperfections in the original may be apparent

Contents

The author and the contributors

Gwynn Davis is Senior Research Fellow in the Faculty of Law, University of Bristol, UK. He has written several books concerning the legal process of divorce, but turned his attention to criminal justice issues in 1985 when, with colleagues at Bristol University, he undertook a preliminary overview of mediation and reparation schemes in England and Wales. The following year the same group of researchers conducted a follow-up study in which they observed the practice of selected schemes at first hand. Mr Davis is currently engaged in a study of the criminalisation of assault.

Heinz Messmer is Research Associate in the Special Research Unit 227 – 'Prevention and Intervention in Childhood and Adolescence', University of Bielefeld, Germany. His main research interest concerns interaction and communication issues in respect of interventions aimed at juvenile offenders. He has published widely on diversion and victim–offender mediation and is the co-author of *Restorative Justice on Trial* (Dordrecht/Boston 1992).

Mark S. Umbreit is Director of Research at the Center for Victim–Offender Mediation – a programme of the Minnesota Citizens' Council on Crime and Justice, Assistant Professor in the School of Social Work at the University of Minnesota, Research Associate at the Center for Youth Development and Research (UM) and Principal Investigator for a cross-site analysis of victim–offender mediation in the US. He also serves as a consultant to the US Department of Justice and as Chairperson of the US Association for Victim–Offender Mediation.

Robert B. Coates was formerly Associate Director of the Harvard Criminal Justice Center, Associate Professor at the School of Social Service Administration of the University of Chicago, and Professor at the School of Social Work at the University of Utah. He is currently a consultant in the criminal and juvenile justice field, Senior Research Associate for a cross-site analysis of victim–offender mediation in the US, and Pastor of a Congregational Church.

Preface

It is rare for a set of ideas to catch on as quickly as did the enthusiasm for victim/offender mediation and reparation in the UK in the mid 1980s; it is rarer still for government to be infected by this enthusiasm, to give pump-priming money, and to contemplate legislation. It seemed, for a while, as if these ideas were to be given a secure institutional form. The position is much less clear today, but this episode (as one may now see it) provides a fascinating subject for academic study since it is not often that one sees ideas emerge, a practice develop, and then support be withdrawn – all within a remarkably short time span. It is now fair to say that, within government circles, mediation and reparation schemes constitute something of a 'dead' subject. But this book is not, I hope, simply a research monograph, although I am proud to have been part of a team which employed such an effective and revealing research method. My intention has also been to use these experiments in order to explore questions central to the principles of criminal justice, thereby stimulating more general jurisprudential and penological debate. Also, for those interested in the politics of criminal justice, the book provides a case study of the ease with which vested interests in the penal system marginalise ideas which threaten basic assumptions.

Two people not named on the title page have made a substantial contribution to the book and I wish they could have had greater acknowledgment than is afforded them here. They are David Watson and Jacky Boucherat, my colleagues on the original research projects. David's theoretical contribution was immensely valuable throughout and some passages are in fact based on earlier drafts of his; his influence pervades the book. Jacky Boucherat was a highly talented researcher, many of her field-notes being an absolute delight; the Exeter and Coventry chapters, in particular, rest on the foundations of her work.

At each of the three centres where we carried out our fieldwork we were given generous access and treated with the utmost courtesy by all staff. It is never easy to be researched, and certainly I would not expect all those engaged on these projects to agree entirely with my analysis, but I am grateful to them for the opportunity which they gave us and for their willingness to share ideas.

I also owe a considerable debt to the Home Office, who funded our two research studies, and especially to Tony Marshall, Principal Research Officer, who was our point of contact throughout. The book will reveal that Tony and I disagree about many things, but it gives me pleasure to acknowledge his unfailing helpfulness and courtesy. I should also like to express my thanks to Pat Thomas and the Trustees of the Nuffield Foundation for their decision to pay for my time spent writing the book.

I have also benefited from the theoretical contribution of Adrian Thatcher, who acted as consultant to the research projects; from the assistance of Nicola Bustin, whose time was paid for by the Bristol University Law Faculty; and from the advice of a perceptive but, sadly, anonymous reviewer. I am also delighted that Heinz Messmer, whose work I have long admired, agreed to broaden the appeal of the book by writing a chapter about mediation and reparation in his country; and that Mark Umbreit and Robert Coates kindly undertook to do the same in respect of the USA.

Finally, I have been extremely fortunate in having the assistance of two highly skilled secretaries: Liz Young, who worked on the original research project; and Pat Hammond, who typed the book in each of its various incarnations. I am heavily indebted to them.

Gwynn Davis

Chapter 1

Introduction

In the 1980s there could be observed, in Europe and North America, a modest revival of some ancient themes in criminal justice. The different strands will take some time to identify, but the overarching and unifying theme was a renewed interest in reparative justice as an alternative both to retributivism and to the various utilitarian projects associated with it. In England and Wales even the Home Office was (briefly) infected by this enthusiasm. Experiments were run, research was commissioned, expectations were raised. In the end, it is possible to argue that nothing much was achieved. Our criminal justice institutions (police; magistrates; the legal profession; the judiciary) were, predictably, unmoved by the prospect of a 'new paradigm' of criminal justice (Barnett 1977; Zehr 1990), whilst government interest vanished in 1986, even as the experimental schemes which it had financed were getting under way. But despite what might appear a disappointing outcome, it will be the contention of this book that these experiments were important, that the vision which they largely failed to realise will endure, and that the shortcomings of our criminal justice system are so profound that further attempts will certainly be made. In part, therefore, this book examines the practice of reparation schemes; but it is also a study of the intractability of our criminal justice institutions.

AN HISTORICAL SKETCH

The recent interest in reparation was largely unheralded, but there is agreement amongst scholars that restitution to crime victims is an ancient institution and that, for most of our history, it has been integral to the practice of punishment (Schafer 1960, p. 5; Maine 1861). Under the Roman Empire, the victim in many cases could choose whether to embark on a civil law suit or, alternatively, initiate criminal proceedings. Maine describes how much crime was dealt with by way of reparation, with the official who 'judged' the dispute behaving in ways not dissimilar to a latter-day mediator (Maine 1861). It would appear from these and other accounts that, for most of our history in the West, non-judicial dispute-resolution techniques have dominated. Schafer (1960, p. 4) describes a general reluctance to seek remedy through the agents of the state. The state had a role, but it was a relatively modest one compared with the dominant negotiation/arbitration models. The more usual pattern was for the offender to offer some form of economic compensation to the victim; if this was accepted, honour was satisfied and the justice process complete.

The gradual evolution, in England, from a system of private dispute settlement to a system for dealing with public 'crime' is described by McAnany (1978). This process coincided with the decline of feudalism and was completed in the fifteenth century. Prior to that time, the responsibility for initiating court action lay with the victim or his family; the court might order restitution, or impose retributive punishment, or it might do both things together. But by the sixteenth century the victim's role in initiating prosecution had disappeared, while restitution as an outcome of criminal proceedings likewise fell into abeyance. The element of private loss or injury was, from that point, virtually ignored, whilst reference was increasingly made to 'the King's Peace' (McAnany 1978).

State control over the processes of prosecution and punishment (and the almost complete displacement of the victim) were probably designed, in the first instance, to gain access to a source of revenue (Schafer 1960, p. 8). Feudal barons and mediaeval ecclesiastical courts had begun this process by requiring offenders to forfeit property to them, rather than to their victims. Subsequently, with the development of the centralised state, the Crown sought to enrich itself through the appropriation of all payments arising from the criminal justice process. The economic interest of the state displaced the economic interest of individuals (McAnany 1978).

The corollary of this transformed view of the nature of 'crime' was that the rights of victims came to be regarded as independent of the criminal law: the obligation to pay damages became an element in the separate realm of civil law, known as the law of torts. The penal law of ancient communities, in which crimes led to an expectation of restitution, has itself been characterised as 'a law of torts'

(Schafer 1960, p. 5), although of course it was not referred to in that way at the time. But from the sixteenth century onwards the courts developed principles which were intended to distinguish between offences against the state ('crimes') and offences against individual rights only. Thus, Blackstone, in his *Commentaries on the Laws of England*, published in 1778, asserted that 'public wrongs, or crimes and misdemeanours, are a breach and violation of the public rights and duties due to the whole community, in its social aggregate capacity . . . since besides the wrong done the individual, they strike at the very being of society' (Book IV, p. 5).

I shall return to this philosophical distinction between public and private wrongs, but first I want to consider what the criminal law of Blackstone's time was really like. For this it is necessary to turn to the accounts of social historians. They tell us that the principal punishments meted out by our criminal courts in the eighteenth century were transportation, whipping, and the stocks, supported by 'a fat and swelling sheaf of laws which threatened thieves with death' (Hay et al, 1975, p. 18). By the middle of the eighteenth century transportation had emerged as the dominant mode of punishment, accounting for some 70 per cent of Old Bailey sentences (Ignatieff 1989, p. 20), but of far greater symbolic significance was the spectre of the hanging tree. Law-makers of the time proved assiduous in enacting an impressive array of particularised capital statutes. In practice, many thieves were sentenced to lesser punishments, or had their death sentence commuted, but even if execution policy was less bloodthirsty than the law allowed, the death sentence hung over every petty thief and criminal law was based on terror, as Hay and his co-authors vividly describe.

Almost all these capital statutes concerned offences against property. In a society marked by a vast gulf between rich and poor, property was deified and protected by 'Albion's Fatal Tree'. Thompson describes how, by these means, the law was able to assume 'the postures of impartiality . . . it was neutral as between every degree of man, and defended only the inviolability of the ownership of things' (Thompson 1975, p. 207). In reality, of course, there was a huge gulf, in terms of wealth and social status, between these 'victims' and their 'offenders'. Perhaps the most dramatic manifestation of the criminal law as an expression of class interest was the Black Act of 1723 (Thompson 1975, passim). This was aimed specifically at protecting the interests of hugely wealthy land-owners against marauding bands of poachers. The Black Act (which probably did not lead to a great many hangings) marked the ascendancy of the doctrine of crude retribution (Radzinowicz 1948, I, p. 77).

It is evident from the accounts of Hay and Thompson that the eighteenth-century criminal law can be understood in terms of class, of property versus non-property, and of symbolic rather than sure retribution. Hay argues (1975, p. 60) that the ferocious – but largely unenforced and unenforceable – penal code of the eighteenth century was designed to protect the ruling class rather than men of middle income. The latter might have preferred a surer system of apprehension, but what really mattered for the landed gentry was the law's reinforcement of their authority. This is a point of crucial importance to this book. The criminal law is as much concerned with authority as it is with property. As Hay puts it, the criminal law legitimised the status quo . . . it was the weapon which ensured that the many submitted to the few (1975, pp. 25–6). This symbolic power of the law was most obvious in the ceremony of the visiting assizes, when the judge's summing-up for the jury and his words to the offender when passing sentence were each taken as opportunities to address the multitude. So it was, according to Hay, that 'in its ritual, its judgements and its channelling of emotion the criminal law echoed many of the most powerful psychic components of religion' (1975, p. 29).

In eighteenth-century England almost all prosecutions were initiated by private persons. Unlike France, we had no state police or state prosecution. The large element of victim discretion which resulted meant that the criminal law was often characterised by displays of mercy and of reconciliation (Hay 1975, p. 40). Precisely because the law expressed the victim's will – that is, the will of the rich, land-owning victim – there emerged many alternatives to prosecution. These included posting a 'bond' not to offend again; paying compensation; and undertaking work for the victim (Hay 1975, p. 41). Alternatively, the thief might simply beg the victim for mercy. According to Hay, many victims 'made the most of their mercy by requiring the pardoned man to sign a letter of apology and gratitude, which was printed in the county newspaper' (p.42). These 'victims' were of course powerful men: their forgiveness reinforced class relationships based upon deference and paternalism.

It is important that we comprehend the significance of Hay's observation (p.56) that the eighteenth-century gentleman accepting an apology from a pauper thief need not have been concerned about the genuineness of that apology: the important point lay in its publicness and therefore in its serving to sustain general belief in the justice of the social order. Thus, in the eighteenth century, apology was tolerated – and even valued – because of the contribution which it made to the symbolic purposes of punishment. It was not private, it was not therapeutic, and it was not heartfelt. This is something to be borne in mind when, in due course, we contemplate the apologies organised by present-day reparation schemes.

In the 1770s there emerged a fundamental shift in the justification for one particular form of punishment – that of imprisonment. This, one might say, was truly a 'new paradigm'. Whereas most forms of punishment – whipping, branding, the stocks – inflicted bodily suffering, imprisonment, on this new conception, was directed at the mind (Ignatieff 1989, p. 46). Prior to 1775 imprisonment was rarely used, comprising only 2.3 per cent of sentences imposed at the Old Bailey from 1770 to 1774 (Ignatieff, p. 15). John Howard changed all that. His *The State of the Prisons* was published in 1777 and in it he set out the programme of discipline – the training of the mind – which he saw as the proper function of the penitentiary. This in turn was refined in Jeremy Bentham's *Panopticon*, published in 1791. According to Ignatieff, the penitentiary promised 'to restore the legitimacy of a legal system that (Howard and his fellow reformers) feared was jeopardised by the excessive severities and gratuitous abuses of the Bloody Code' (p.79). The penitentiary was intended to achieve moral reclamation, implanting 'guilt and compunction in working class consciences' (Ignatieff, p. 213). In order to produce guilt, the treatment had to appear to be humane. Solitary confinement was the answer, offering 'a punishment so rational that offenders would punish themselves in the soundless, silent anguish of their own minds' (Ignatieff, p. 213). As Ignatieff demonstrates, penitentiaries manifestly failed in their reforming intent, as well as being bitterly cruel in the imposition of solitude upon prisoners, but they were functional to the extent that they symbolised the imposition of rational order and discipline in the face of looming social breakdown. The new prison regime therefore commanded the support of the propertied classes, being, as Ignatieff explains (p.213), a hopeful allegory of class relations in general and therefore well able to survive its practical failure.

It can be seen from Ignatieff's account that the rise of what Cohen has termed 'the more economically and politically discreet prison sentence' (Cohen 1985, p. 25) reflected a tendency to punish harder, this in turn being fuelled by an enthusiasm for the utilitarian projects of reform and deterrence. Cohen also endorses Foucault's thesis (1975, passim) that when the state turned to imprisonment, punishment became reasonable: 'Interest was transferred from the body to the mind – a coercive, solitary and secret mode of punishment replacing one that was representative, scenic and collective' (Cohen 1985, p. 25). Furthermore, because imprisonment was a standardised form of punishment, it was more readily controlled by the state. If Cohen's analysis is correct, it would seem that the experiments which I shall describe in this book were conducted in a most unpromising climate. For Cohen is one of the leading proponents of the thesis that we are witnessing a continued expansion of the power of central authority even as, it is feared, social cohesion is being lost (see also Cain 1988). Also, despite a loss of faith in utilitarian punishment, there still appears little viable alternative to the discreet prison sentence. Reparation schemes, however flawed in their conception, can be regarded as attempts to move in the opposite direction, that is, to develop forms of criminal justice which are visible, which will promote social cohesion, and which at the same time will not be dominated by the central authority (in other words, by police and courts). It is hardly surprising, viewed in this light, that the counter-vailing forces proved too strong.

A PHILOSOPHICAL SKETCH

The distinction between public and private wrongs, referred to by Blackstone, has become a settled and dominating feature of the justice process. Criminal law is characterised by the central role of the state: the state is victim; the state prosecutes; the state punishes (Zehr 1985). In civil law, on the other hand, it is assumed that private citizens are in conflict; the outcome is expressed in terms of compensation. The division of law into these two strands has had major consequences for the outcome of criminal proceedings and for the treatment, within those proceedings, of the victims of crime. As McAnany puts it, 'the victim's right of recourse was lost with the emerging field of tort' (McAnany 1978). One reason for this is that the victim was viewed as the embodiment of revenge and therefore as likely to prove hostile to the project of achieving social re-integration of the offender. The emergence of rehabilitative thinking was one manifestation of a utilitarian perspective, and from this perspective (whether the utilitarian was concerned with reform of the individual offender or general deterrence) the victim was regarded as having little to contribute. Attention was focused on possible *future* crimes which the judicious use of punishment was intended to deter. Restitution might be one way of adding to the overall burden placed on offenders, but was not an essential component given that the objective was to administer a punishment sufficiently severe to deter others. As a consequence, growing interest in individual reformation and general deterrence coincided with a loss of interest in the victim – and, specifically, a loss of interest in reparative outcomes.

This, broadly, remains the position today. State control over the justice process is considered necessary in order to achieve uniformity of outcome. It is also defended as flowing from our awareness of the broadly social cost of criminal acts. The intrusion of what may appear to be elements of civil law into the criminal justice process is, in general, resisted by the legal profession, it being feared that the introduction of compensation will divert attention from the primary objectives of the criminal justice process, namely, punishment and deterrence (Campbell 1984). It is also feared that victim compensation would re-introduce various anomalies and inconsistencies which the civil/criminal law distinction is intended to overcome (Wasik 1978). As a result, compensation has remained a peripheral and relatively insignificant part of the criminal process . . . 'a quickie civil suit tacked on to a basically criminal procedure, appropriate only to very straightforward cases and relatively menial crimes' (Campbell 1984). This, certainly, was the view of the Dunpark Committee, when it considered the scope for reparation within criminal justice in Scotland (Dunpark 1977). Dunpark was dismissive of all arguments in support of reparation save that of 'doing something for victims'. The Committee did not regard compensation as a criminal justice measure, but rather as a 'short-circuit civil action' which they were prepared to concede might be linked to the criminal process. As Campbell (1984) observes, Dunpark regarded reparation as quite distinct from criminal justice; it was acceptable provided it did not disrupt court timetables or prove unduly expensive, but only because it conveniently permitted criminal charges and civil suits to be settled at the one time.

It is consistent with the marginal status of reparation that there has been fierce resistance to the idea that reparative acts (whether or not these take a material form) might have a bearing on the punishment imposed by a court. Enoch Powell, in a forceful contribution to this debate, has argued that 'the whole concept of crime and the law is undermined if the satisfaction or indemnification or appeasement of the private citizen injured through a crime is treated as capable of eroding or aborting the reaction of the state to injury offered to itself . . . the idea that a crime might not be punished, or ought to be punished less severely, because the object of the crime forgives or accepts satisfaction proffered by the perpetrator is of great destructive potential' (Powell 1985). Powell's attack is centred on any tendency to regard private reconciliation as appropriately influencing the court's response to 'crime' – which by definition is committed against the state. But he does not directly address the question of whether 'justice' might be geared, wherever possible, towards restitution and reconciliation. Nor does he deal with the implicit challenge posed by legal anthropologists such as Nils Christie to the present practice of hiving off certain kinds of harmful behaviour and calling them 'crime', whilst allowing much other harmful behaviour to be regarded as a civil wrong, or no wrong at all as far as our courts are concerned.

Underlying this difference of view, it might be said, are competing conceptions of what 'justice' might look like in response to, say, theft or assault. In considering this we are bound to be influenced by our familiarity, through the media, with the present impersonal, professionally dominated criminal proceedings, and also by our understanding of the reasons why we punish. One value of the anthropological perspective is that it enables us to view the familiar with fresh eyes, to the point where we may even regard it as bizarre. As Priestley (1977) has observed, the criminal justice process is invoked when one person (the offender) fails to observe the legally protected rights of another (the victim). But what then happens is that the state interposes itself as the victim, while the concerns of the person who suffered the hurt are effectively excluded: the process of trial and punishment makes no attempt at aid or succour. Instead, there is, as Priestley puts it, 'a most astonishing attack on the person, the personality and the property of the offender'.

If reparation is normal and retribution bizarre, as Priestley suggests, it seems inappropriate that reparation be developed in such a way as to serve the interests of our present court system. Howard Zehr (1985) has observed that reparation is often 'sold' in the language of punishment, whereas what is needed is 'a new language' in which justice is no longer seen in terms of exacting the appropriate level of retribution. Reparative justice requires the court to consider what the offence meant to the victim and, secondly, to consider what the victim regards as being necessary in order to put the damage right. The underlying aspiration has been well described as that of 'seeing the offence not as separated from life, but as an element of social behaviour' (Frehsee 1987, p. 139, quoted in Messmer 1989). According to Messmer, the object is to seek reconciliation which is 'true to life and intuitively plausible'. This is likely to prove an arduous task, as Messmer's own research makes clear, but the rewards are correspondingly great. In Messmer's terms these amount to the abandonment of abstract demands for punishment by the state and, secondly, the withdrawal of 'unnecessary educational influences' – in other words, reform initiatives.

Barnett (1977) has likewise argued that our entire criminal justice system might have a reparative base. According to Barnett, 'crime is an offence by one individual against the rights of another. The victim has suffered a loss. Justice consists of the culpable offender making good the loss he has caused'. Barnett proposes, therefore, that we abandon retribution entirely; indeed, as far as he is concerned, retributivism is fading before our eyes . . . 'we are witnessing the death throes of an old and cumbersome paradigm, one that has dominated Western thought for more than 900 years' (Barnett 1977). Apart from the over-simplification (there has been more than one 'paradigm', as we have noted), there are several reasons why such a view might be considered exaggerated. The first is that the rights infringed by the offender are possessed not just by the individual victim, but also by other citizens. The offender's social relationship with the victim has been damaged, but so too has his relationship with other citizens (Davis et al, 1987; Watson et al, 1989). The offender's behaviour implies lack of concern for, and perhaps denial of, the victim's rights in his or her property and possessions; but his actions may also be taken to imply lack of concern for the rights of other citizens; *their* security has likewise been damaged. This is why the social value of any changed attitude on the part of the offender is under-estimated if it is presented as a change towards the victim personally. Reparation (whether or not this takes a material form) which reassures an individual victim of the offender's changed attitude towards his or her rights should also reassure others who possess the same rights. This is why, for example, it would be inappropriate for a victim to determine the extent of his or her 'own' offender's obligation to make reparation. The interests threatened are, to some extent, held in common; others are therefore entitled to a voice in decision-making. Any compensation judged to be due might go to a *particular* victim, but the reassurance is an intangible shared with other right holders.

Another reason for reservation is that critics of retributivism (and of prisons in particular) sometimes fail to take account of the symbolic purposes of our justice apparatus to which reference has already been made. Courts and prisons may fail to meet their ostensible goals, such as rehabilitation or deterrence, but still have symbolic value. The symbolic purposes suggested by Priestley (1977) are as follows: defining the boundaries of acceptable behaviour; articulating a secular account of good and evil; and promoting social solidarity and cohesion. It is possible of course that reparative justice might serve those self-same purposes, but it cannot do so if it is conceived as belonging to the private realm.

It follows from this that we need to review the standard opposition between civil and criminal law. This has indeed been attempted by those commentators who have been prepared to treat compensation as a form of punishment (Schafer 1960; McAnany 1978; Campbell 1984; Watson et al, 1989). As Campbell puts it, compensation may be regarded, not as 'a conceptual cuckoo in the criminal law nest, but as a possible penal objective which can, without undue theoretical difficulty, be incorporated into the notion of criminal justice and even into the concept of punishment itself'. According to Campbell, reparation fits the philosophical consensus concerning the defining features of punishment, namely, the intentional authorised infliction of suffering on an offender for an offence. This is also the position adopted by Schafer, who refers to 'the restitutive concept of punishment' (1960, pp. 117–122). Such thinking has not penetrated very far in criminal justice circles, but it is not counter-intuitive: the appropriateness of offenders compensating for the harmful consequences of their criminal acts is even more obvious than in the case of civil wrong, to which no moral stigma may attach (Campbell 1984). As Campbell makes clear, this need not be viewed in terms of the *replacement* of punishment by reparation, but rather as the integration of the two.

A possible counter to this way of thinking (also identified by Campbell) is to define punishment according to the intention with which it is inflicted. Thus, one might make punishment retributive by definition, if the sole object is to inflict pain. But 'punishment' is commonly acknowledged to have several purposes – deterrence, reform, containment – in addition to retribution. Why cannot reparation be added to the list, so that it becomes a further – indeed, perhaps the main – object of punishment? Interestingly enough, justice expressed in terms of making good appears perfectly compatible with several elements of retributive theory, although less compatible with utilitarian approaches based on notions of general deterrence. Both restitution and retribution are 'act-based' (McAnany 1978); that is, they are concerned with the harm done in that one case, rather than with extraneous factors contributing to the offender's character or social circumstances. Both are generally proposed in a form which acknowledges the moral significance of individual autonomy. Furthermore, they are each species of distributive justice; the root metaphor in each case is that of justice as balance, the object being to restore the distribution of rights which existed prior to the offence. One may conclude from this that, far from being in opposition, the return of reparative thinking was made possible, in large part, by the re-emergence of retributive theory as the justification for punishment. In other words, the relative demise of utilitarianism, the re-discovery of the victim, and renewed interest in reparation, all fit together rather well. Or as McAnany puts it: 'the fit is so nearly exact that the reinvention of the victim in criminal justice and the return of retribution as the primary explanation of why we punish appear to be manifestations of the same social movement' (McAnany 1978).

There are, however, two important reasons why to regard reparation as one element (even the key element) in punishment may appear problematic, or deficient. The first is that to subsume reparation within punishment works well enough for financial or work-based reparation, but not so well for those aspects of reparation which are non-material and cannot be coerced. Non-material reparation is important because the harm done by an offence is never confined to damage to a person's body or property; it also involves damage to a social and moral relationship, however tenuous. This arises because victim and offender are related in the sense that they are both citizens, presumed to be law-abiding, in a society in which the victim is acknowledged to have rights in his or her person or possessions. The offence gives the victim good reason for fear for his or her rights in future. Except where the event was accidental and non-negligent, the offender's action implies lack of concern for, or perhaps even denial of, the victim's rights. So 'reparation' cannot be solely material; if it is to be adequate, it must include some attempt to make amends for the victim's loss of the presumption of security. The offence has undermined the victim's belief in the existence of moral standards held in common. This means that it has threatened his or her moral relationship with the offender by providing grounds for review of mutual obligations based on trust. The presumption of security and of common values can only be restored by some effort to reassure the victim that his or her rights are now respected; in other words, by some sign of attitude change – or, alternatively, some indication that the offence was 'out of character' (Watson et al, 1989).

The other difficulty about the attempt to reconcile reparation and retribution has to do with the weakness of the 'justice as balance' formulation which underpins both paradigms (Lukes 1973). Social inequality might be said to threaten the moral basis of both retribution and material reparation. 'Security of possessions' (MacCormick 1978) is controversial in that the degree to which we think this ought to be protected depends on our view of the justice or otherwise of the distribution of resources within society. It could be argued that the selection of offending behaviour brought to the attention of our courts, and even legal definitions of what constitutes 'crime' in the first place, reflect the values and protect the interests of a dominant social group. Indeed, it may be supposed that our essentially retributive system of justice has developed in response to this heterogeneity and stratification, it being unrealistic to expect much in the way of 'reparation' from the somewhat unrepresentative and generally impecunious group of citizens who come to the attention of our criminal courts.

But while it is important to acknowledge the problematic nature of 'justice as balance', one of the strengths of the reparation case is that it positively demands that we place the offence in context – that context being the financial and other social circumstances of the victim and offender. There will be many instances where the distribution of resources, skills, and opportunities may be so unequal that material reparation is not a practical proposition – and, even if it were, to impose restitution upon offenders who, by almost any yardstick, find themselves at the bottom of the heap would offend rather than satisfy our sense of justice, undermining the moral message which it was the court's intention to convey. Retribution may be imposed without these broad issues of social justice being addressed at any stage, whereas that is almost inconceivable under a reparation-based system. This is confirmed by the clear offender-orientation of the reparation schemes which we studied (for which see Chapters 3 to 5). It is also the experience in the USA: McAnany observes that 'while restitution as a theory clearly has the victim in mind, its primary interest has remained the offender'. This is not to suggest that the interests of the offender should subvert those of the victim. But it is appropriate in any 'justice' system to be concerned for the offender: as Adrian Thatcher has observed, care for offenders is as important as care for victims (Thatcher 1991).

THE COURT PROCESS

No analysis of possible alternative ways of thinking about justice, even one as brief and preliminary as this, would be complete without some analysis of the way our present court system works. It is because these public forums violate most of our intuitive notions of what constitutes a just process that the impetus for reform persists. Perhaps the most obvious example of this lies in what Roberts has referred to as 'the narrow concept of relevance' applied within criminal proceedings (Roberts 1979, p. 21). Issues to which no legal rules apply are not justiciable, no matter that they may give rise to a profound sense of grievance. There is no scope at all for the redress of *emotional* hurt. As Roberts puts it, 'a precise issue . . . is separated from any larger complex of relations between the two disputants and dealt with in isolation from other aspects of their relationship' (Roberts 1979, p. 21). The legal process is not much concerned with explanations; the 'meaning' of the offending behaviour (for victim as well as offender) is not normally registered by the court. If, for example, there is a prior personal relationship, this is unlikely to affect the way in which an offence is viewed. To the extent that the background to the offence does intrude, through the probation officer's social enquiry report or the defence solicitor's plea in mitigation, it is orientated solely towards the offender; there is no attempt to present the whole picture (Wright 1982, p. 241).

A second, related criticism is that victim and offender are denied effective participation in the court process. Baldwin and McConville (1977, p. 83) report that 'one of the most immediately striking findings to emerge from our interviews with defendants, all of whom were legally represented, was their profound sense of non-involvement in, if not complete alienation from, the legal process in which they had been concerned'. Blumberg (1967) has likewise observed that 'the defendant is outside the network of intimate relationships that comprise the court'. Furthermore, 'the specific objectives of the other actors are seen as by no means concordant with those of the defendant. Indeed, their interests may well conflict with his'. An example of such conflict, powerfully conveyed by Baldwin and McConville, arises from the court's expectation that defending solicitors and barristers achieve a high proportion of guilty pleas. These authors describe the pressure on defendants to plead guilty, given the inducement of a lesser charge or the promise of a lesser sentence. They noted twenty-two cases in which the guilty plea arose from an explicit plea bargain, and twelve in which the defendant pleaded guilty, although expressing doubts as to whether what he did was criminal. The latter category included crimes of violence in which the defendant claimed that a distorted account of the incident was presented unchallenged to the court: 'The defendant commonly felt that, had an accurate picture of the circumstances surrounding the wounding or assault been given, he would have been acquitted or, at least, given a much less severe sentence. Each defendant said he had been told by his barrister that he would be convicted at trial, that it was dangerous to contest the case and that matters such as self-defence ought not to be put forward' (Baldwin and McConville 1977, p. 64). The 'justice' which emerges from these accounts appears not so much retributive as economic, or administrative. The image of comparative justice is sustained in the courtroom, but in the vital preliminary negotiation other considerations prevail. Evidence such as this makes a very strong case, not just against plea bargaining, but against forms of justice which take little or no account of the 'stories' of victim and offender – stories which might lead to the offence being re-described.

It can readily be argued, on the other hand, that our guilty plea system is an administrative necessity. Auerbach refers to the calculation made in the USA that if a significant proportion of criminal cases went to trial, the administration of justice in American cities would disintegrate . . . 'Plea-bargaining barely kept the system afloat, at the cost of an insidious dilemma: if legitimacy depended on adherence to the legal forms of a fair trial, necessity required their circumvention in order to process the deluge of criminal complaints' (Auerbach 1983, p. 122). This might appear a serious weakness in the case for reparative justice delivered through our criminal courts: how can we possibly find time for victim and offender to tell their stories so that the scale and nature of reparation may be determined? This is a question to which I shall return. Reparation is likely to remain a feeble plant indeed under a guilty plea system, or in the absence of victims.

That reparative justice requires *participation* is in fact a large part of its appeal. Nils Christie (1977) contrasts the vitality of tribal justice with 'the greyness, the dullness, and the lack of any important audience' which characterises Western legal systems. Bottoms and McClean likewise came to the conclusion that 'for the most part, the business of the criminal courts is dull, commonplace, ordinary and after a while downright tedious' (Bottoms and McClean 1976, p. 226). Christie suggests that the main reasons for this are that our forms of justice are inaccessible; the parties are peripheral to the process; and the state has taken over the accusatory role of the victim. This is a loss to every single one of us, in Christie's view, but it is especially a loss to the victim: 'the victim is so thoroughly represented that she or he for most of the proceedings is pushed completely out of the arena, reduced to the triggerer-off of the whole thing. She or he is a sort of double loser; first, vis-à-vis the offender, but secondly and often in a more crippling manner by being denied rights to full participation in what might have been one of the more important ritual encounters in life. The victim has lost the case to the state' (Christie 1977).

While the victim loses the right to be heard, we *all* lose in the sense that we are unable to identify with the justice process. It is no longer psychologically satisfying – for the victim, the offender, or for other citizens. We are often told, in newspaper accounts, of the detached stance adopted by offenders as they are sentenced. But what other response is possible when you are the subject of such a calculated assault from professional punishers? Primitive emotion is distrusted, so we aim at objectivity through a highly refined legal process – the high point of this being, in most instances, the striking of a bargain between lawyers. This, it may be supposed, has no psychological value for any of the participants (Balint 1951). The case for reparative justice rests, in large part, on the supposition that highly significant, highly contentious events in people's lives should not be resolved by a boring, mysterious process.

THE RETURN OF REPARATION

A renewed interest in 'reparation' – whether as an integral part of criminal justice or an alternative to it – may be traced to the USA, and in particular to the Mennonite religious communities whose faith led them to espouse the principles of atonement and reconciliation (Umbreit 1985). The first Victim Offender Reconciliation Project (VORP) was begun in 1978 in Elkhart, Indiana and the model was soon replicated in many other towns and cities, the majority of these projects conforming to the original VORP model which strove to achieve both financial compensation and reconciliation between victim and offender. These schemes generally operate independently of the criminal justice process; in most instances the offender will already have been sentenced by the court; the mediators are concerned with victims and offenders equally (Coates and Gehm 1989).

Similar developments took place over the same period in Canada. In 1974 the Ministry of Correctional Services began to link decarceration with help to victims. The Ministry supported a project in Kitchener, Ontario, which had been proposed by the Mennonite church (Peachey 1989). The original conception linked several key themes, many of which continue to resonate in the debates surrounding reparation in the UK. These include: maintenance of 'community'; decarceration; reconciliation; reformation; moral accountability; victim involvement; and low cost (Rock 1986, p. 177).

In the wake of these US and Canadian initiatives the idea of reparation, in its various guises, found its way into European discussion of criminal justice. It has generally been viewed as a possible *alternative* to criminal prosecution (rather than as an element within the justice process) and has commonly been applied only to juvenile offenders. Aside from developments in England and Wales, considered in Chapter 2, there have been reparation initiatives of various kinds in Germany (where innovative research has also been done – see Messmer 1989 and Chapter 9); in France; in Norway; and in Finland.[1]

It should not be assumed that these projects share a common purpose, that the institutional arrangements are similar, or that the mediators' practice is consistent. Diversity is inevitable given the constellation of ideas which have led to this renewed interest in reparation from almost every corner of the political spectrum. Two ideas, in particular, have been influential.[2] One is the development of *labelling theory* and *interactionism* in the 1960s through the writings of criminologists such as Becker (1963) and Lemert (1967). This contributed to an undermining of the category of 'offender' and demanded a re-appraisal of long-established beliefs about the causation of crime and the appropriate treatment of offenders. The second is the Durkheimian notion of the *inevitability* of crime. If we accept that the boundaries of 'crime' are elastic, and that laws will always be broken, we may be free to abandon notions such as the 'war against crime' in order to concentrate on doing something useful in the situation we have.

Other more immediate factors favourable to the development of reparation include a growing disenchantment with a prison system which, it is claimed, achieves none of its original purposes except immediate containment and which, furthermore, is almost certainly criminogenic. This view appears to be accepted by the UK government whose recent pronouncements stress the virtues of 'punishment in the community' (Home Office 1988 and 1990). But whilst it seems generally to be accepted that imprisonment has little to commend it beyond containment and that alternatives need to be found, there is also considerable scepticism about programmes of individualised treatment or rehabilitation. This rejection of crime treatments which are rooted in notions of individual pathology has been characterised as a movement 'back to justice'. Reparation, on some accounts, is part of this. Given that prison reinforces criminal careers, there is attraction in the idea, not just of alternative punishments, but of a new way of understanding what 'justice' might be.

Nevertheless, retributive thinking runs very deep in our culture: it is not going to be abandoned entirely. One empirical research finding which has proved useful in advancing the reparation case is the discovery that victims do not, in general, endorse the call for more severe penalties (Shapland et al, 1985). This in turn makes it feasible to pursue another objective which, in many people's minds, underpins the case for reparation, namely, to reduce the level of pain delivered at the hands of our criminal courts (Christie 1977 and 1982, passim). A belief in punishment as *utilitarian*, and delivery of that punishment by representatives who are distant from victim and offender in terms of social status and values held in common, both tend, in Christie's terms, to create a climate which is conducive to high levels of pain delivery. If it is understood that victims are not necessarily affronted by decisions to punish less, and if it is acknowledged that what courts do, for the most part, is deliver fresh pain, then it may be feasible to develop forms of justice which are not pain-based.

Criminological interest in victims has either concentrated on

possible ways to alleviate victim distress and suffering in the aftermath of crime (Shapland et al, 1985), or else, as noted above, victims
have been viewed as an unwelcome constraint upon the humane
treatment of offenders. The former preoccupation has manifested
itself, in England and Wales, in the introduction of a system of
compensation orders in criminal proceedings; in greater priority
being given to such compensation orders; in the creation of the
Criminal Injuries Compensation Board which provides state funds
for victims of violent crime; and in the whole 'Victim Support'
movement (Shapland et al, 1985). Renewed interest in reparation
suggests a possible redefinition of the post-crime relationship between victim and offender. The rhetoric of reparation emphasises
victims at least as much as offenders. This has led McAnany, for
example, to conclude that 'restitution . . . has ridden on the coat-
tails of a larger phenomenon in criminal justice: the reinvention of
the victim' (McAnany 1978). But, as Laurie Taylor has observed,[3]
concern for the victims of crime is far from being a new phenomenon: it is the favourite refrain of the 'law and order' lobby which uses
the *image* of the victim in order to argue for more severe punishment
of offenders. There is a risk that the reparation movement may use
victims in a not dissimilar way: that is to say, it too may evoke the
image of the victim (the ignored, bypassed victim in this instance) in
order to achieve greater credibility when seeking to promote new
ways of dealing with the offender (see also Walklate 1989, pp.
125–126).

   Another powerful idea underpinning recent North American and
European interest in reparation is the quest for 'community' and for
communitarian justice, outside the institutions of the state. The
search for justice without law has been chronicled by Auerbach
(1983, passim). Many of these initiatives have been co-opted by the
state, but the search for 'alternatives' has been very persistent. Cohen
likewise refers to the attractions of 'simplicity, intimacy, equality and
security – the alleged small town virtues of pre-industrial rural
America; a romantic yearning for "direct", "traditional", or even
"tribal" forms of conflict settlement and dispute resolution' (Cohen
1985, p. 35). According to Cohen, 'this ideology . . . has come to
dominate Western crime-control discourse in the last few decades'
(Cohen 1985, p. 116). An image of justice delivered in stateless
societies has indeed been imported into Western criminological
debate. There are of course many aspects of tribal justice – ostracism,
shaming, physical retaliation, resort to sorcery – which it may be

thought undesirable to replicate, although it might be contended that these supposedly alien elements do indeed figure in our system, even if we prefer not to acknowledge the fact. However, there are other elements of tribal justice – such as the go-between, transmitting messages from one disputant to another, or the mediator, actively coaxing the parties towards a settlement (Roberts 1979, p. 26) – which, viewed from a distance, present an appealing contrast to the impersonality of our ways of delivering justice.

Linked to the notion of community, there is the idea that certain disputes are mistakenly and damagingly dealt with as crimes, thus ignoring the history of the conflict and denying its inter-personal elements. For some commentators, indeed, it would appear that 'dispute' is a kind of pre-crime, or crime in embryonic form (Launay 1985; Marshall 1985). Crime is what happens when disputes are not dealt with in proper, communitarian ways. The same commentators (e.g. Marshall 1988) sometimes advance an alternative formulation in which they appear to suggest that the 'crime' and 'dispute' labels should be abandoned altogether in favour of the generic category of 'trouble'. Courts, it is argued, are unable to respond to disputes or 'trouble' because they are constrained by procedural delay, by rules of evidence which prevent them enquiring into matters which the parties themselves deem to be significant, and by the criminal sanctions which they impose (Chinkin and Griffiths 1980). It would seem therefore that 'neighbourhood justice' (of which reparation is but one part) has the potential to relieve pressure on busy courts; to deal with 'trouble' in ways which address the true meaning of the conflict; and to stop disputes becoming crimes.

As is well known, the ability of neighbourhood justice to deliver what it promised has come under sustained attack. Tomasic has identified some eighteen assumptions underpinning the case for mediation as a method of dispute resolution in the US – all of them questionable, in his view. Among the most central are the beliefs that neighbourhood justice centres provide easier access to the legal system; that there is such a thing as a sense of 'community'; and that mediators 'represent' the community and share its values (Tomasic 1982, p. 215). Cohen likewise identifies 'the idealistic flaw of trying to base a social control ideology on visions derived from other societies . . . the content of these visions may be historical and anthropological nonsense – underplaying the paternalism, the fixed lines of authority and the arbitrary nature of justice. Conservatives forget the high degree of conflict and disorder. Both sides tend to

ignore the implicit threat of violence which often lay behind the
submission to community or informal justice' (Cohen 1985, p. 121).
Cohen disparages this as the 'folk museum' version of justice in
which ideas of integration, mutual help and good neighbourliness lie
dormant but waiting to be revived. Auerbach is similarly pessimistic.
He contends that neighbourhood justice centres in the USA contra-
dict all the prerequisites for informal justice: communities played no
part in their design; legal institutions hover over the programmes;
and virtually every project receives its cases from the court, thereby
serving as an exit rather than an entry point to justice. He observes
that 'alternative dispute settlement served as a tenacious metaphor for
missing elements of community in American cities; but there was
little in urban life to sustain it as a functioning process' (1983, p.
134). Instead, these agencies came to serve the interests of the state
legal apparatus in promoting the efficient processing of criminal
complaints.[4] Auerbach's conclusion, therefore, is that these initiatives demonstrate the futility of the attempt, by agencies of the state,
to establish justice without law.

Despite these gloomy prognostications, it is inevitable and right
that there should be resistance to our centralised, professionally-
dominated court system. Neighbourhoods may be weak, but if we
are content to regard courts as a kind of private club where lawyers
practise mysterious arts, then we lose any sense of a relationship
between formal justice and the conflicts in our own lives. The person
who has identified the loss which this entails and who has written
most imaginatively about it is Nils Christie (1977; 1982, passim;
1986). Christie argues that our industrial society does not have too
many conflicts: it has too few. The depersonalisation of social life
means that people have limited information about one another. This
in turn makes it harder to cope with conflict. As Christie puts it, 'not
only are professionals there, able and willing to take the conflict
away, but we are also more willing to give it away' (Christie 1977).

It is important to understand that Christie is seeking to emphasise,
rather than to undermine, the importance of public forums. In that
sense his vision is neither 'alternative' nor 'abolitionist' (Dünkell and
Rössner 1989). His position is that we need more trials, rather than
fewer, but that the nature of the trial process needs to be transformed. This runs counter to the strong tendency, perhaps most
evident in the UK, to regard courts as inevitably retributive, and
reparation as necessarily voluntary and extra-legal (FIRM 1988).
Christie's vision may be Utopian, but at least he places reparation at

the heart of the justice system. Voluntary reparation performed in social work offices may have therapeutic value, but it presents no challenge to the practice of courts, whilst reparation which is said to be voluntary but which seeks to *influence* courts is bound, as we shall see, to collapse under the weight of its own contradictions.

PLAN OF THE BOOK

In Chapter 1 I have reflected upon the history of some of the main theoretical concerns contributing to a revival of interest in reparation justice. Chapter 2 reviews political and practical developments in England and Wales, utilising our own preliminary survey of reparation schemes. Chapters 3 to 5 are the heart of the book, offering a detailed analysis of the practice of reparation in England and Wales, based on direct observation of three sharply contrasting initiatives. Chapter 6 to 8 review this research evidence, identifying the dominant themes and also those themes which were conspicuous by their absence. Chapter 9 is written by Heinz Messmer: as well as reviewing the history of victim–offender mediation in Germany it offers an account of Messmer's own research into mediation in the aftermath of fights between juveniles. Chapter 10 is written by Mark Umbreit and Robert Coates and provides an overview of research into victim–offender mediation in the USA. In Chapter 11 I consider ways in which reparative principles might be more fully integrated into the practice of criminal justice.

NOTES

1 For an overview of these developments see Marshall and Merry (1990).
2 Both noted by Laurie Taylor in an address to an early conference on reparation in the UK, organised by the Forum for Initiatives in Reparation and Mediation at Chelsea College, London, on 15.4.85.
3 FIRM conference, 15.4.85: see note 2.
4 For an account of similar developments in the field of matrimonial dispute, see Davis (1988).

Chapter 2

Developments in England and Wales

Interest in reparation in England and Wales has its roots in two distinct reform movements. The first of these, which one might characterise as 'the victim movement', reflects a widespread concern for the material and emotional well-being of the victims of crime. The second, which one might term 'the offender movement', seeks to re-cast our justice system in a variety of ways, some of the main themes being anti-punitiveness; responsibility and involvement; expiation; and rehabilitation.

Concern for crime victims has itself led to three kinds of initiative. First, there was the introduction of the Criminal Injuries Compensation Board in 1964. This provides state funds to compensate the victims of violent crime. It is independent of the criminal justice process and may therefore be regarded as akin to other 'welfare' payments made by the state in response to a category of citizen need (Campbell 1984). It is in fact the major source of financial compensation for crime victims (Shapland et al, 1985).

Secondly, there have been steps taken to introduce financial compensation by offenders as an element within criminal proceedings. The Criminal Justice Act 1972 introduced a general power to order compensation for any offences resulting in any kind of loss to any identifiable victim (Shapland et al, 1985). This provision is now embodied in s.35 of the Powers of Criminal Courts Act 1973. It was strengthened by s.67 of the Criminal Justice Act 1982 which enabled courts to impose compensation as the sole penalty for an offence, and by the Criminal Justice Act 1988 which required courts to give reasons for *not* awarding compensation in cases where it had been requested. As noted in Chapter One, the introduction of compensation into criminal proceedings has not been without its theoretical and practical difficulties. For the most part it is afforded only a minor role, the predominant judicial attitude being reflected in Lord Widgery's pronouncement that 'A compensation order made by the [criminal] court can be extremely beneficial as long as it is confined to simple, straightforward cases and generally cases where no great amount is at stake'.[1] This had likewise been the view of that notably conservative body, the Dunpark Committee (Dunpark 1977) who considered that compensation orders must not interfere with 'the smooth running of our criminal courts'. Dunpark likewise observed that one disadvantage of the compensation order was that it 'introduces a foreign element, namely, reparation for civil wrongs, into the administration of criminal law' (6.06). In general it is fair to say that the practice of compensation in English criminal courts has not gone beyond the Dunpark prescription, which was that it 'must be confined to clear and simple cases, because criminal procedure is not designed to facilitate the adjudication of complicated or disputed claims for compensation' (6.06).

A third form of assistance available to crime victims is that offered by the national network of victim support schemes. The National Association of Victim Support Schemes was established in 1979, following which there was a rapid growth in the network of affiliated schemes. This was followed by an element of state funding, but the schemes continue to be staffed by trained volunteers. They take referrals from the police, shortly after a crime has been reported, and then visit the victim at home in order to offer what support and assistance they can (Reeves 1989).

These, then, were the three obvious manifestations of 'the victim movement' in the early 1980s. In the minds of many, the development of reparation schemes was likewise aimed at improving the lot of crime victims. But in this instance, even more obviously than in relation to court-ordered compensation, a new service for victims carried clear implications for the treatment of offenders. Indeed, many proponents of reparation were not especially interested in victims: for them, 'reparation' was the means whereby offenders were to be offered education and the hope of exculpation, rather than be required to submit to useless pain. These ideas were introduced in Britain in the 1970s, an early example being a speech by Philip Priestley to the Margery Fry centenary proceedings in Birmingham in 1974. The vision of reparative justice being advanced at that stage was heavily influenced by models then being developed in the USA (Wright 1981; Harding 1982). These American ventures contained elements of financial compensation and so were acceptable both to retributivists and to those who preferred to emphasise the educative and cathartic possibilities of reparation. At the same time, government interest in reparation was stimulated by a perception that these schemes might assist in reducing – or at least stabilising – the cost of courts and prisons in the face of an ever-rising number of prosecutions. In other words, it was hoped that reparation might contribute to the official policy of 'diversion' (Davis et al, 1988). It was probably for this reason above all others that, in 1980, the National Association of Victim Support Schemes was approached by the Department of Health and Social Security to ask if NAVSS would establish some experimental juvenile reparation projects to run alongside victim support: the funding offered was far in excess of the then total government grant to NAVSS (Reeves 1989).

NAVSS declined such a role because it wished to maintain its own clear identity, but it is noteworthy that a service so clearly identified with the victim interest should have been selected as the focal point for initiatives in reparation: it suggested a remarkable coalescence of interests. Despite its initial reluctance, NAVSS began to assume the role of information service for the embryonic reparation projects which got off the ground around this time (Reeves 1989). Meetings of interested parties were held on a more or less regular basis. Out of these grew the Forum for Initiatives in Reparation and Mediation (FIRM), formed in 1984, which soon attracted more attention and support than NAVSS, the organisation which gave it birth.

Most of the early practice initiatives in the UK took place under the aegis of the probation service. The first court-based reparation scheme was a 'special project' run by the South Yorkshire probation service from November 1983 for an experimental period of three years. Also in 1983 the West Midlands probation service obtained a grant from the Cadbury Trust which enabled it to employ Martin Wright to carry out a feasibility study in Coventry (Harding 1989). Wright recommended an American-style 'Earn-it' scheme under which unemployed offenders would be found work in order that they might recompense their victims. This proposal aroused opposition within the probation service and the eventual form of the Coventry Reparation Scheme (for which see Chapter 4) could hardly have been more different from that envisaged by Wright.

Since the probation service is an organisation which has always concerned itself exclusively with offenders, probation sponsorship suggested that reparation was likely to be developed in ways which promoted the offender interest – either through education and reform, or through diversion and mitigation. This, of course, was not the impression created by the early links with NAVSS. The National Association of Probation Officers expressed reservations for this very reason (NAPO 1985), and certainly the difficulties at Coventry gave some indication of the problems that could arise, but otherwise it is fair to say that the question of conflicting purposes and competing constituencies was not addressed. Reparation was afforded the reception common to many abstract ideas which lack precise definition: it was welcomed by almost everyone (for an illustration of this, see Marshall and Walpole 1985).

In 1984 reparation was given the imprimatur of government approval when Leon Brittan, then Home Secretary, made an enthusiastic speech to the Holborn Law Society. Brittan identified the main benefits of reparation as follows: 'First, through reparation, the criminal justice system can concentrate its attention on the individual victim whose interests must never be ignored. Secondly, the principle of reparation can be used to ensure that the wider interests of society are better served, and thirdly, nothing is more likely to induce remorse and reduce recidivism among a certain, all too numerous, kind of offender than being brought face to face with the human consequences of crime' (Brittan 1984).

Also in 1984 the Home Secretary announced that money was to be made available to fund a small number of reparation projects on an experimental basis. This announcement attracted enormous interest and there was fierce competition for the limited amount of money available. In February 1985 the government announced that £200,000 would be spent over two years on reparation projects in Cumbria, Leeds, Wolverhampton and Coventry. The Cumbria scheme was to test reparation in conjunction with a police caution; Wolverhampton and Coventry were to examine reparation as an adjunct to other disposals for low-tariff offenders in the magistrates court; and the Leeds scheme was to be based in the Crown Court, where it would explore the potential for diverting high-tariff offenders from custody.

The projects sponsored by the Home Office were each to be evaluated by independent researchers. At the same time David Watson and I were commissioned by the Home Office to conduct a preliminary review of all forms of reparation then being undertaken in England and Wales. We only had twelve months in which to do this and so were bound to rely heavily on schemes' own accounts of their practice. We asked the co-ordinators of all the projects listed in the Home Office report *Bringing People Together* (Marshall and Walpole 1985), plus some others which we heard of along the way, to complete a questionnaire and to send us any relevant literature. From a total of 41 questionnaires sent out, we had 33 replies, 24 of them from schemes which attempted to mediate between the offender and his or her own victim. We also visited seventeen schemes in order to talk to organisers and their staff, to peruse records, and to meet representatives of related professional groups. This preliminary enquiry provided a useful introduction to the subject, prior to our undertaking the much more searching investigation of three reparation schemes in 1986/7, for which see Chapters 3 to 5.

At the time of our initial survey, several 'schemes' identified by the Home Office were little more than *statements of intent*, or, alternatively, modifications of existing practice introduced by individual probation officers acting on their own initiative. Some of these projects soon changed their priorities and mode of operation; others folded altogether; whilst yet others, such as Coventry, gained further financial support. It seemed to us that the various schemes could be sub-divided into: (i) those which operated prior to the prosecution decision being taken, or in conjunction with a non-prosecution disposal such as a police caution; and (ii) court-based or post-sentence schemes.

All pre-prosecution schemes were concerned solely with juveniles. In so far as they engaged in victim/offender mediation, this was usually in conjunction with a caution, as a kind of enhancement of it. This would normally be agreed with the police in the course of negotiating a non-prosecution disposal (see Chapter 3). Once a decision to caution had been taken, this would not then be reviewed, even if the young offender declined to 'make reparation', or if such reparation as was offered proved unsatisfactory to the victim. Nevertheless, as we shall see, the relationship between the offender's willingness to undertake reparation and the police decision not to prosecute could in practice become blurred.

Court-based schemes dealt mainly with adult offenders and were generally linked to the magistrates court. Most were run by the probation service, with much of the workload being carried by accredited volunteers. With the exception of Leeds, Coventry and Wolverhampton, all funded by the Home Office, only two court-based schemes had any full-time paid members of staff. In terms of their relationship to the court, they could be sub-divided as follows:

1. Schemes in which the possibility of reparation was identified prior to any court appearance and mediation between victim and offender attempted prior to the hearing (see Chapter 5).
2. Schemes in which mediation was attempted on adjournment (see Chapter 4). This group could be further sub-divided in that there were some courts where the probation officer took the initiative in attempting to mediate between victim and offender following a routine social enquiry report request; other courts adjourned specifically in order that the reparation option might be explored.
3. A very few post-sentence schemes. Mediation might be undertaken following the interim disposal of a deferred sentence; or in the context of Intermediate Treatment; or as a condition of a probation order; or, more rarely, it might form one element in a community service order.

SELECTION CRITERIA

I now turn to an examination of the criteria upon which reparation schemes based their choice of cases. The first point to make – a deceptively simple one – is that all schemes agreed that an admission of guilt by the offender was necessary before negotiation between victim and offender could begin. In other words, the obligation to make reparation had to be accepted. But this is where reparation undertaken *alongside* the formal processes of prosecution and punishment can present an immediate problem. The difficulty is simply that an informal acknowledgement of responsibility need not give rise to a guilty plea in court. We heard of one case in Leeds where a meeting between the offender and a representative of the scheme was followed by a not-guilty plea: this caused consternation at the time, the judge taking the view that the defendant's case had been compromised.

The offender focus

When schemes were invited to outline their selection criteria, they did so with reference to offender characteristics, rather than by referring to any measure of victim need or desert. The tendency to refer to offender characteristics was so deep-rooted that most practitioners appeared not to recognise this orientation, let alone question it. The administrative arrangements adopted by most schemes tended to confirm that the victim interest was not at the forefront of their thinking: the timing of the intervention was inevitably related to a threatened prosecution or a pending court appearance. We heard that one reason why some victims were reluctant to take part was that they were approached so long after the offence had been committed that they were no longer concerned about it. Thus, the Leeds scheme told us of one case in which 'the mediator tried to re-awaken (victim)'s feelings of anger, just in case, but didn't succeed'. It is true that both pre-prosecution and court-based schemes referred to the needs of victims, but the method of selecting cases and the clear focus on the offender's pending or threatened court appearance suggested that victim needs were in fact secondary.

The tariff

For the most part selection of cases was determined by consideration of the tariff. Most schemes focused on minor offences and on offenders with a relatively modest criminal record. The most common offences were theft, assault, criminal damage and (more occasionally) burglary. Crimes of violence, sexual offences, and serious and/or persistent offenders were generally ruled out. The only exception was the Leeds scheme which was geared to serious offences and high tariff offenders. This was partly 'to test out ideas behind reparation with people who had committed a serious offence' and partly because 'we needed to get the finance from the Home Office – it was a selling point'. In practice even Leeds was prepared to deal with cases where the offender was not, in fact, at risk of imprisonment.

The focus on minor offences reflected the presumed link between reparation and diversion. Because serious offences cannot be diverted from prosecution, and because very serious offences cannot be diverted from imprisonment, it was assumed (not only by police, magistrates and judiciary, but by the staff of reparation schemes) that reparation was inappropriate as a response to serious crime. I shall develop this point in subsequent chapters, but suffice it to say here that the presumed link between reparation and diversion imposed a debilitating and unnecessary limitation on the practice of many reparation schemes.

Personal or corporate victims

Many schemes had given thought to the question of whether mediation should be attempted in cases where the victim was a corporate body such as a large store, a factory, a local council parks department, or an educational institution. Some probation-based schemes were reluctant to attempt reparation in such cases, their reservations being in line with NAPO policy: 'We have noted the possibility of reparation being made to large chain stores, companies etc. Whilst recognising that it can be viable, we are . . . doubtful whether the unequal distribution of resources and power between the two participants make equitable resolution and mediation possible or even desirable' (NAPO 1985). However, the main reservation concerning reparation to corporate victims arose from the fear that this negotiation would have less 'meaning' for the offender. Blagg's research at Corby had been influential here and was referred to by several schemes. He observed that reparation to corporate bodies (usually in the form of apology to a representative) was often unsatisfactory 'due to the restrictive scope for reconciliation and understanding' (Blagg 1985). The problem as Blagg saw it was that a representative could not be expected to feel 'the range of confused personal feelings and hurt emotions' which one might hope to address in mediation. As a result, the offender might experience the meeting as further punishment. This indeed was the reaction of some of the juvenile offenders whom Blagg interviewed at Corby: 'they were punished by an authority figure, they were powerless to prevent the process, they acquiesced' (Blagg 1985). In some instances this may be the price which the offender has to pay for securing diversion. The pressure (or the inducement) which operates in these circumstances means that the offender cannot be regarded as a free agent.

The decision to engage in mediation only with non-corporate victims tells us much about the objectives of reparation schemes – and especially about their wish to confront the offender with a distressed or angry victim in the hope that this will promote attitude change and affect future behaviour. A representative is less likely to provoke contrition – although quite capable, one might have thought, of negotiating restitution. In fact schemes adopted differing policies in relation to this issue. As will become apparent in Chapters 3 and 5, the Exeter and Totton schemes were quite prepared to mediate between offender and corporate victim. Other schemes have 'real' victims rather than representatives.

The importance of a prior personal relationship between victim and offender

It has been estimated that some 39 per cent of assault victims are assaulted by persons known to them (Shapland et al, 1985, p. 108).

O'Brien, in a survey of victims in the Gloucester area, found that almost a quarter of her sample of victims knew the offender well, whilst a further quarter had had some previous contact or knew the offender by sight (O'Brien 1986). It was held by the organisers of some reparation schemes that offences committed in the context of a continuing relationship lent themselves most naturally to mediation and reparation. An experiment run by the Metropolitan Police actually stipulated that victim and offender should have been known to one another prior to the commission of the offence.

The prior personal relationship criterion was not adopted with anything like the same rigour at other centres. Of far greater significance was the *seriousness* of the offence, with reparation being deemed appropriate only for those at the lower end of the scale. As a consequence, a minor shoplifting might be accepted for mediation, whilst serious violence against someone with whom the assailant was in daily contact would be deemed 'high tariff' and therefore inappropriate (Nelken 1986).

PROBLEMS OF IMPLEMENTATION

I have said enough to indicate that reparation schemes in England and Wales experienced considerable difficulty in evolving a coherent philosophy and practice. They also – even in the enthusiastic early days before the Home Office withdrew its interest and support – experienced many practical problems. Applying for funds; gaining and maintaining co-operation with outside agencies; securing cases; seeking to influence the court – all proved extremely frustrating and time-consuming. The main problem experienced by several schemes was that of gaining a sufficient number of cases. Various explanations were offered as to why, in the first year or two, there was so little to show for all the effort put in. For the most part the reasons given boiled down to difficulties with the parent agency (usually probation); or with the police; or with the court. I consider each of these in turn.

Lack of resources/other demands within the agency

Most reparation schemes are run by the probation service. In these circumstances the co-ordinator is usually a probation officer. Many of these officers found that little or no allowance was made for the

time which they needed to devote to this new venture in order for it
to succeed. Alternatively, there may have been an attempt to seek
additional funds in order to employ specialist staff, but these fund-
raising ventures could themselves be extremely time-consuming,
with no certainty of eventual success. The problem in essence was
that reparation was viewed as a development of the probation task
and therefore not as something which merited the allocation of
additional resources. Volunteers were expected to bear the brunt of
this additional work-load. From the point of view of the co-
ordinators, this proved to be an unrealistic expectation. They found
that considerable time was taken up in the selection, training, and
support of volunteers. This was so even where a scheme had very few
cases. Southampton, for example, was referred two cases in its first
nine months, but volunteer meetings continued to be held on a
regular basis, calling for a considerable time commitment from the
probation officer in charge.

With or without volunteers, schemes were inevitably dependent
to some degree on the co-operation and support of colleagues within
the probation service, both at main grade and management level.
This was partly a question of freeing time in order that the officer
concerned might devote time to reparation, and partly of having
sufficient interest and enthusiasm to make the appropriate referrals.
By and large the organisers of the various schemes were disappointed
by the reaction of their probation colleagues. Pressure of work, lack
of understanding, plain inertia – all were mentioned as contributing
to this lack of response. Even if they accepted the idea as a good one
in principle, probation colleagues tended to regard any new venture
as creating more work for them. Also, unless they were themselves
imbued with the excitement of creating something new, they did not
have sufficient interest in the scheme to remember to think about it
in relation to their own work.

There were also frequent references to upper management in-
difference to reparation. This was apparent, for example, in the
highly restrictive offence categories which were imposed as much
from within the probation service as by the police or court. Another
limitation which we observed was that of permitting only one officer
to engage in reparation – even though this was undertaken in the
course of his routine social enquiry work and so could hardly be
considered a 'scheme' as such. This evidence of institutional defen-
siveness within probation no doubt reflected management's need to

curtail demands upon the service's resources. In these circumstances the strategy which is likely to provoke least discomfort is that of maintaining the present pattern of resource allocation.

The NAPO line on reparation

Probation officer ambivalence or hostility towards reparation arose in part from the stance adopted by their national association, although it is fair to say that the initial hard line was subsequently modified. The original NAPO view was that, whilst they were not against reparation in principle, they opposed the use of current probation resources in the development of reparation schemes because this would dilute the service's concern for offenders (NAPO 1985). Accordingly, probation officers in some areas were reluctant to co-operate with the embryonic reparation schemes run by their colleagues – which meant that they failed to refer potential cases. Ann Garton's interim report on the Leeds scheme noted a mixed response among probation officers in the city . . . 'Many were doubtful about the advisability of diluting concern for offenders with that for victims, and anxious, too, about long-term resource implications' (Garton 1986). The co-ordinator of the Coventry scheme told us that 'one of the main problems has clearly been the effects of NAPO policy on any mutually beneficial relationship being developed between the scheme and the probation service. This means few referrals from this quarter and some problems when cases are referred to the scheme and for social enquiry report at the same time'. Totton likewise reported having received only five referrals from probation officers in their first year of operation – this because probation staff were ambivalent about the scheme.

Securing co-operation from the police

Reparation schemes are inevitably dependent upon the co-operation of the police. Pre-prosecution schemes are totally reliant on the police for their supply of cases. Those court-based schemes such as Totton (see Chapter 5) which attempt to mediate prior to the initial court appearance are in a similar position. Even court-based schemes which operate on adjournment require the co-operation of the police if they are to gain access to victims. It would appear that the police response varied both by region and by rank. Several pre-court schemes reported difficulty in securing sufficient (or any) referrals from the police. It emerged from our investigations with police officers that they regarded reparation schemes as being mainly concerned to help the offender; the police responsibility, on the other hand, is to protect the rights of victims. In some areas this protectiveness towards victims led the police to be wary of cooperating even with victim support schemes (described by one senior police officer as 'a far more sellable concept') lest victims regard them as an intrusion. Reparation was viewed as much more problematic – that is, a service intended *for* offenders and therefore likely to place an additional burden on victims.

Despite these doubts and reservations, some schemes experienced wholehearted co-operation from the police. South Yorkshire reported 'full co-operation from police and prosecuting solicitors' in gaining access to prosecution files. In the interim report prepared by the Rochdale scheme it was said that 'liaison and co-operation with the local police have been efficient and amicable, requests for information being dealt with quickly and correctly'. But the Rochdale experience is instructive in that while the mediators gained the support of upper management within the police force, they encountered considerable scepticism on the part of main grade officers. The latter tended to regard reparation as a means whereby offenders could 'con' victims, a soft option, social work nonsense – and so on. Senior police officers whom we interviewed at other centres appeared well aware of the sceptical, even derisory attitude adopted by some of their main grade colleagues towards reparation schemes. They recommended, in fact, that the co-ordinators should liaise only with senior officers, by-passing the cynical lower ranks.

Gaining the co-operation of the court

The main difficulties experienced by court-based schemes were in getting their probation colleagues to recommend the reparation option to magistrates and, secondly, in getting courts to ratify such recommendations as were made. Part of the problem lay in alerting magistrates to the existence of the scheme. It was suggested to us at some centres where reparation had been available for a year or more that most magistrates remained unaware of it. Another difficulty was that magistrates were sceptical about reparation attempted prior to an initial court appearance because they saw it as restricting their sentencing options, or at least putting them under pressure to deal more leniently with the offender than they might otherwise have done.

Finally, some magistrates lacked enthusiasm because they understood the scheme's mitigatory intent and so tended to be sceptical of the offender's motives in meeting the victim, or indeed in making any form of 'reparation'. These various difficulties had considerable influence upon the practice of reparation at Coventry and Totton, as I shall describe in Chapters 4 and 5.

THE HOME OFFICE

Some months after the Home Secretary announced government sponsorship of four reparation schemes, the Home Office produced a discussion paper (Home Office 1986) which was to prove a watershed in the development of reparation in the UK. This was not an especially coherent document, and its review of the scope for reparation – and specifically of the relationship between reparation and the criminal courts – reflected all the uncertainty and confusion of the time. But what it did reveal, quite astonishingly given the forms of reparation which the Home Office had committed itself to sponsoring, was that government interest in this subject was largely centred on the possibility of an additional court penalty – a 'reparation order' – which would provide an alternative disposal for minor offenders. This was of little interest to most practitioners within the various embryonic reparation schemes. Such a clash of expectations, when it was revealed, dealt a fatal blow to the development of reparation in England and Wales. In order to understand why this should be it is necessary to look a little closer at the discussion paper itself.

In its preliminary account of the projected benefits of reparation, the discussion paper appeared to reflect the thinking of project organisers, although it placed greater emphasis upon victim reassurance and material reparation and rather less upon mitigation, or upon therapeutic aspirations in relation to offenders. It asserted that:

> The thinking behind the schemes which have sprung up, first in the United States and more recently in this country, is that sensitive mediation (usually a face to face meeting between the victim and offender in the presence of a third party with a view to agreeing reparation) between offender and victim, where both are willing, can bring benefit and reassurance to the victim and can help the offender to face up to the human consequences of his behaviour and think twice before repeating it. Where material

reparation is desirable and possible, it can be arranged, but even where it seems unnecessary, the process of mediation may, it is argued, be of great value.

(para. 5)

The discussion paper also considered the timing of any mediation, although it was evident that the main issue concerned the extent to which reparation should be brought within the ambit of the court. The paper referred to two ways in which this might be done under existing powers: first, in the context of a deferred sentence; and secondly, as one element within a probation or supervision order. The former option was thought to have been 'considerably circumscribed' by an Appeal Court decision, although, reading reports of this decision, it is difficult to discern why it should circumscribe anyone. The Lord Chief Justice had merely asserted, without supporting argument, that 'It will, one imagines, seldom be in the interests of justice to stipulate that the conduct required (upon deferring sentence) is reparation by the defendant'.[2]

Reparation ordered as one element within a probation order was considered a viable option, but it was thought that probation (or the equivalent 'supervision order' in relation to juveniles) should involve a wider programme for the offender, going beyond a specific act of reparation. Furthermore, it would be unsatisfactory if offenders whom the court would otherwise have punished 'less elaborately' – say, by a fine – were to be placed on probation simply in order to attract the reparation condition.

This led the authors of the discussion paper to consider the need for a separate 'reparation order' – an option which they clearly favoured. It also emerged, however, that the Home Office (at least at that time) regarded such an order as inappropriate 'for those convicted of more serious offences and at risk of the most severe penalties' (para. 18). If agreed tasks were not performed satisfactorily, the offender should be returned to the court. The discussion paper also assumed that reparation should be managed by the probation service, in conjunction with 'voluntary bodies' (para. 23). Finally, whatever institutional arrangements were made for the development of reparation, these were 'unlikely to justify the allocation of new resources' (para. 27).

So, a court order, with the court retaining oversight of the reparation imposed, and no additional resources. The reaction to this document from the various reparation schemes was, as might have been anticipated, almost uniformly hostile. Indeed, perhaps the most remarkable aspect of the discussion paper was the extent to which it revealed a failure of communication (or of co-ordination) between two branches of the Home Office. There appeared to have been an almost total lack of liaison between, on the one hand, the policy division responsible for the discussion document and, on the other, the Research and Planning Unit (in particular, the Principal Research Officer with responsibility for this area, Tony Marshall who had overseen the sponsorship initiative). This pump-priming money had been provided for a juvenile panel concerned to achieve *diversion*; and to probation-run schemes principally concerned to promote expiation, catharsis, and mitigation. The only point of convergence between the Home Office and the initiatives which it was meant to be sponsoring for experimental purposes was a pre-occupation with the offender and a corresponding willingness to employ victims in pursuit of the offender interest. That aside, there was an almost complete mis-match between the policy question posed by government and the experiments which it hoped would provide an answer.

Something of the flavour of this failed meeting of minds can be gathered from an account of a seminar on reparation held at the Institute of Advanced Legal Studies on 23rd July 1986 (Nelken 1986). Nelken reports that most contributors to the discussion had fundamental worries about whether reparation was at all compatible with the current justice system . . . 'The attack was led by many of the judges and magistrates present, and Sir Jack Jacob commented afterwards that the "sentencers" had scored a number of goals in attacking the idea of introducing reparation into the criminal justice system. In fact, no contributor to the discussion defended the Home Office approach in its present form'.

According to Nelken, magistrates and judges argued that there were already enough options available to the court, including com-pensation orders. To take account of whatever reparation had been undertaken would lead to inequity in the treatment of offenders . . . 'More broadly, since the goals of sentencing were pre-eminently concerned with deterrence and denunciation, they could not be subordinated to the achievement of reparation and reconciliation between particular offenders and victims. For their part, advocates of reparation insisted that they too did not see it as supplanting the existing sentences available to the court nor even as representing a new mode of disposal . . . . Experience of reparation schemes had demonstrated that victims were typically interested in receiving an apology and overcoming the psychic and emotional scars of crime, far more than in the sort of direct compensation which could be measured and standardised as a disposal technique for the court'. As Nelken observes, this discussion revealed competing conceptions of what criminal justice ought to be about. The question of the relationship between reparation and the courts remained unanswered: should reparation be completely separate from the court; should it become part of the armoury of the court; or (a possibility barely imagined by any of those present) should it come to dominate the proceedings of the court?

The result of these differences in outlook was predictable. Reparation schemes (including the ones which the Home Office was paying for) uniformly rejected the idea of a reparation order. They did not object, it would seem, to reparation performed under the rather murky incentive of a sentencing discount, but they did not want it to be imposed by a court. The schemes' umbrella organisation, FIRM, responded to the effect that 'participation must be felt by both parties to be voluntary and non-coercive' (Reeves 1989). FIRM preferred to regard reparation as something separate from the justice process, 'so that the opportunity for reconciliation between victim and offender would be entirely unconstrained' (FIRM 1986).

Evaluation of the FIRM response is complicated by the fact that it was largely written by Tony Marshall, the Home Office Research Officer who had been responsible for handling the reparation initiative. Marshall was a prominent member of FIRM. In due course he was seconded from his job at the Home Office to become that organisation's first full-time Director. He had no sympathy with the Home Office objective of tying reparation to the sentencing process. To this extent the lack of congruity between experiment and policy objective can be traced directly to Marshall. Because he was at odds with his paymasters, he presided over a widening gulf between the objectives of government and the practice of reparation schemes. His was indeed a pivotal role: he was the midwife of the reparation schemes; he was responsible for commissioning the research which would monitor their effectiveness; he became Director of FIRM and drafted FIRM's responses to the various Home Office policy documents, including the crucial 1986 discussion paper. Subsequently, having taken up his post with FIRM, he continued to co-ordinate the various research efforts and he also drafted the eventual composite Home Office research report on reparation schemes (Marshall and Merry 1990).

The publication of this latter document was delayed for as long as possible by the Home Office, who also demanded substantial amendments to Marshall's original draft. They had little sympathy with his defence of the more ephemeral virtues of victim/offender mediation. As far as the Home Office was concerned, 'reparation' had taken a direction which it had no interest in pursuing. Accordingly, it delayed publication of Marshall's report for some two years, well beyond the point when it was likely to attract political interest. Indeed, when *Crime and Accountability* eventually appeared the Home Office did not even consider it necessary to issue a press release. Reparation had disappeared from the political agenda. It had originally been supposed that the reparation order might be introduced as one element of the 1986 Criminal Justice Bill, but that proposal had foundered when schemes' hostility to the proposal became known. The official reason given was that the Home Office was awaiting the results of the reparation experiment, but in reality Home Office officials had come to appreciate that any reparation initiative coordinated and researched by Marshall was most unlikely to produce findings upon which the government would wish to act.

The Home Office meanwhile had honoured its commitment to the four reparation schemes which it had undertaken to sponsor for two years, but had then withdrawn. This did not mean that these and the various other initiatives folded; some, such as Coventry, attracted the support of a charitable trust or foundation, while in many areas the local probation service continued to allow their staff (and volunteers) to spend time on reparation. But the Home Office had moved onto safer ground. In October 1986 the Home Secretary announced substantial additional funding for victim support schemes. This marked a retreat from the difficulty and controversy associated with reparation and a reversion to the safe political project of 'doing something for victims'. My colleagues and I had direct evidence of this loss of official interest in reparation when we proposed a further study, not of reparation schemes as such, but of the scope for reparative outcomes across the range of prosecutions in our criminal courts. The Home Office turned down our application (this was in 1987) on the basis of 'the remoteness of the central ideas from current policy concerns'.

This did not mean that the Home Office had given up all thought of promoting reparation, but it soon emerged that it had adopted a highly circumscribed view of the form which this reparation should take – a view wholly at odds with that of Marshall and FIRM, and contrary to the research findings which Marshall had produced. The government Green Paper, *Punishment, Custody and the Community* (Home Office 1988) placed the emphasis upon 'punishing offenders in the community'. The value of reparation was extolled in this context, but when it came to explaining *why* reparation might be of some value, confusion reigned. Paragraph 1.4 stated:

> Another feature of the Government's policies has been the rapidly developing emphasis given to the position of victims. Requiring offenders to make some recompense for the injury, loss or damage they have caused to individuals or the community is one way to bring home to them the harm they have done and the serious view which most of us take of their actions . . . The Government considers that compensation to individuals and reparation to the public should be an important element of punishing offenders in the community.

A series of non sequiturs such as this reminds one of Cohen's dictum that what the social control system does is invariably accompanied by much talk (Cohen 1985, p. 157). These 'good stories' as Cohen calls them are meant to tell us what the system thinks it is doing, but the stories do not hang together . . . 'The language which the powerful use to deal with chronic social problems like crime is very special in its banality. Invariably, it tries to convey choice, change, progress, and rational decision-making. Even if things stay much the same, social-control talk has to convey a dramatic picture of break-throughs, departures, innovations, milestones, turning points – continually changing strategies in the war against crime' (Cohen 1985, p. 157). In this case the solution suggested was 'punishment in the community'. This would contain three elements: (a) some deprivation of liberty; (b) steps to reduce the risk of re-offending; and (c) compensation 'to the victim and the public' (Home Office 1988, para. 3.8). This highly conventional pot-pourri of the traditional aims of criminal justice was to take the form of a new sentence, a 'supervision and restriction order', which might include elements taken from the following list: compensation to the victim; community service; residence in a hostel or other approved place; prescribed activities at a day centre or elsewhere; curfew or house arrest; tracking an offender's whereabouts; plus other conditions, such as staying away from particular places (Home Office 1988, para. 3.27).

It can be seen therefore that, at least as far as official thinking was concerned, reparation had resumed its former place at the margins of criminal justice. Perhaps it was never intended that it should do more than this; it may simply have been social control talk. Later in 1988, the then Home Secretary, Mr Douglas Hurd, issued notes of guidance to courts in relation to compensation for criminal violence. Mr Hurd reminded the courts that one way to bring home to offenders the harm which they had inflicted upon their victims was to order compensation. This led *The Times*, in a leading article, to assert that: 'the separation of the civil from the criminal consequences of a violent act was a false dichotomy. It only encouraged the mistaken impression that there were two distinct aspects to the matter, an offence against the law being different from an offence against the individual. The Home Secretary is right to insist they are the same. He is also right to propose that compensation should, in certain cases, be the only criminal penalty, and should always take precedence over a fine' (*The Times*, 21.09.88). Unfortunately, government emphasis upon compensation orders, appropriate though this may be in many instances, does not have the fundamental effect which *The Times* seemed to imagine. Criminal proceedings retain their focus upon the offender; the tenor of these proceedings is unchanged: the state is responding to an offence committed against itself; compensation remains peripheral. This much is acknowledged in the same *Times* leader, when, in a concluding paragraph, it is asserted that the purpose of a compensation order 'is primarily to demonstrate to the criminal his personal responsibility for damage. If it is to do that, it has to hurt.'

Faced with such time-honoured sentiments dressed up as reform measures it is little wonder that Tony Marshall and FIRM prefer other stories – the 'reconciliation' and 'new approach to conflict resolution' stories. Unfortunately, as I shall describe, the practice of most reparation schemes was determined by their (largely unacknowledged) diversionary and mitigatory objectives. That is why I have written this book. I was depressed by the lack of imagination reflected in the Home Office view of the scope for reparation, but I do not accept that the official research document provides either an accurate description or a convincing explanation of the practice of reparation schemes in this experimental phase.

NOTES

1 Regina v. Kneeshaw [1975] Q.B.57.
2 Criminal Appeal Reports [1984] pp. 211–214; Crim.L.R. [1984] pp. 504–506.

Chapter 3

The Exeter Youth Support Team

The Exeter Joint Services Youth Support Team (YST) is a multi-agency project which has been in operation since 1979. It aims to pool the resources of police, probation and local authority social services in order to provide a range of support services for young people, plus a co-ordinated response to juvenile crime. When fully staffed the team consists of a senior social worker and three other social workers, one with responsibility for Intermediate Treatment; a police inspector, two sergeants and a police constable; and a probation officer. According to the team's own literature, they wish to 'test a model of juvenile liaison', a central purpose of this being 'to encourage through inter-agency co-operation the diversion of young offenders from prosecution'. One of the alternatives to prosecution offered by the team is their reparation scheme, started in 1980 'with a view to assisting the young person to integrate with his (or her) community in a positive way, through taking steps to put wrong things right by methods which will hopefully benefit the offender, victim and community as a whole'.

STAFF DUTIES AND ACCOUNTABILITY

In addition to contributing to the decisions of the YST, social workers within the team are expected to provide Social Enquiry Reports to the juvenile court and to carry small caseloads of children and their families. The probation officer likewise has to attend the juvenile court, has a limited caseload of older children on supervision orders, and spends one day a week with his parent agency. The police members of the team also have additional responsibilities: for example, they co-ordinate the response to all child abuse and child sexual abuse cases (of which there are many). The police are also expected to perform duties which have nothing to do with the YST, such as helping in 'special operations', including the policing of strikes, royal visits and football matches. The sergeant with responsibility for organising reparation is also, as it happens, a member of the police 'defensive weapons team'.

The YST share one premises, but they are not so much a team as a collaborative enterprise involving three separate agencies, with YST staff being clearly identified with their parent agency and remaining accountable to senior staff within those agencies. So the police members of the team are accountable to the Inspector; social workers to the senior social worker; and the probation officer to his 'senior' in the Exeter probation service. Thanks partly to the division of work, and partly to differences of ethos between parent agencies, there can in practice appear to be two teams operating side by side, one of which comprises social workers and the probation officer, and the other, the police.

ORGANISATION

Although the YST acts as a referral point for non-crime matters, it is mainly in business to develop a co-ordinated response to juvenile offending in Exeter. Referrals are made via a '121a' form, completed by the arresting officer, which contains basic information about the offence and may also include reference to the offender's attitude at time of arrest, an account of his or her criminal record, and an opinion as to the appropriate disposal. A '121a' will be followed in due course by a full police file which includes offender and witness statements and some more information about previous offences.

A 'liaison meeting' determines the offence disposal in each case (prosecution, or one of a variety of non-prosecution responses). The discussion is led by the Inspector (or, in her absence, by a police sergeant) and is also attended by the senior social worker and the probation officer. A decision might be deferred in order for one of the social worker members of the team to undertake 'a pre-liaison visit' (PLV) to the young person and his or her family. In that case the social worker prepares a written report and (usually) attends the liaison meeting at which the case is next considered. In determining the response to the offence, the objective, according to the team's own literature, 'is to consider all possible alternatives to prosecution, diversion being the overriding principle, but the decision is balanced against the need to consider the victim as well as the offender and whether it is necessary to use reinforcement of a caution or a warning'.

POSSIBLE OUTCOMES

Possible offence disposals range from 'No Further Action' to prosecution. NFAs are generally reserved for such minor transgressions that it is doubtful, in fact, whether a criminal offence has been committed (in one example, boys found playing with matches in a park). Alternatively, a decision might be taken to 'NFA' an offence where the juvenile concerned is denying guilt and there is insufficient evidence to secure a conviction (as with Steven Rouse, in Case One below).

A formal *caution*, delivered by the Inspector and citable in court, is the most common decision arrived at by the group. This attracts the greatest degree of consensus of all the possible disposals. For most juvenile offenders aged 14 or over, this is their starting point on the tariff. That being the case, there is a reluctance on the part of the police, in Exeter as elsewhere, to deliver repeat cautions for similar offences. In these circumstances the liaison meeting will look to some 'reinforcement' of the caution. One such reinforcement is a requirement that the offender attend a so-called Induction Group, which meets weekly for six weeks. The object of this is to encourage young offenders to review their offending behaviour.

Alternatively, the offender may be asked to make 'reparation'. This may be done by means of a letter of apology (lower tariff); or by apologising to the victim face to face (higher tariff); or by undertaking work-based reparation, such as gardening, this being considered the most onerous of all the possible alternatives to prosecution.

Whilst all the above reinforcements of the basic caution, including the various forms of reparation, are offence disposals agreed by the team, they are voluntary in the sense that they are undertaken after the caution has been administered. Typically, an offender's willingness to participate is assessed in the course of a pre-liaison visit. The formal request (or decision, as it may appear to the youngster concerned) is put by the Inspector immediately upon delivery of the caution. It is unknown for anyone to refuse at this stage.

THE REPARATION SCHEME

The reparation scheme was set up in 1980 and is run by a police sergeant and police constable, both members of the YST. They make the arrangements for whatever form of reparation has been agreed at the liaison meeting. This includes asking the victim whether he or she is agreeable to such reparation being performed. As already indicated, reparation is regarded as one rung on a pre-prosecution tariff: in that sense it is very clearly offender (and punishment) orientated. The object is to arrive at an appropriate response to a criminal offence.

The YST are reluctant to arrange financial compensation from offender to victim. They may well encourage the offender to make good the victim's financial loss, but will not take responsibility for ensuring that this is done. The team institute reparation to both individual and corporate victims. Indeed, corporate victims predominate because of the large number of shoplifting offences. In most of these cases the stolen goods have already been recovered; accordingly, the reparation arranged by the scheme will usually take the form of an apology to the shop manager.

THE RESEARCH

It will be clear from the above account that the Exeter YST regards reparation less as a good in itself than as a means of assisting the case for diversion from prosecution. In order to understand the place of reparation within the overall scheme of things we decided to observe each stage of the process, up to and including any reparation undertaken. We attended liaison meetings at which referrals were discussed; accompanied team members on pre-liaison visits when offenders were assessed; observed the delivery of formal cautions; and attended the various stages of the reparation process. We were with the Exeter Youth Support Team for three days per week over a three month period, beginning mid February 1987. In this time we sat in on twenty-eight liaison meetings; accompanied workers on twelve pre-liaison visits; observed the delivery of three cautions; and followed seven cases which involved some form of reparation.

THE CASES

I shall now give a brief account of four cases observed in the course of our time spent with the Exeter YST. These have been chosen because, in my judgement, they give a good indication of the team's approach to reparation. We did not observe *all* discussions and meetings held in respect of each case. I have employed pseudonyms throughout.

Case One

Jason Coombes and Steven Rouse
Jason and Steven (12 and 14 respectively) have been charged with stealing 90p from an elderly woman's house while they were out carol-singing. Steven is denying guilt, so it is intended to prosecute him. Jason has admitted the offence. He had previously stolen from his own home, shoplifted, and made hoax emergency phone calls.

First liaison meeting

At this meeting, following the suggestion on the file from the police. officer who had read the evidence, it is agreed to consider 'Caution and Reparation' for Jason. It is hoped that once he's been cautioned, he may supply a witness statement sufficient to enable Steven to be prosecuted. The case is referred for a PLV in order to discover whether Jason's version of events will clarify Steven's guilt and, secondly, to discover whether 'reparation' is appropriate. Jason's social worker, present at the meeting, is asked to undertake the PLV. She argues at this stage that the team should look to the possibility of a letter of apology rather than a meeting, as the latter could be too demanding for a child who is already quite disturbed. A PLV is also agreed in the case of Steven, to discover whether he is still denying the offence.

Pre-liaison visit to Jason Coombes

Jason lives in a Children's Home and has done so for some months. His parents had insisted he leave home after he had repeatedly stolen money from them. Jason is interviewed in the presence of a residential social worker.

The social worker undertaking the PLV, Donna, explains to Jason that on this occasion she is visiting him specifically to talk about the offence. She asks him to describe the whole incident.

He and Steven, he said, went carol-singing. At the house in

question, they were left waiting at the door whilst the woman went to get her purse. They noticed money left in an ashtray by the telephone. Encouraged by Steven, Jason took the ashtray with the money in it, threw the ashtray away, and shared the money with Steven (about 90p). Steven saw someone approaching, gave the money back to Jason, and then denied all involvement in the offence.

This happened when Jason was on weekend leave, staying with his parents. His mother had insisted that he go to the woman and apologise: on his mother's suggestion, he bought the woman a box of chocolates and they both went to see her. Since she was out, Jason, again at his mother's instigation, wrote a note of apology on the bag containing the chocolates. The note and chocolates were left at the woman's door.

This story leaves Donna in something of a quandary. She has come, in part, to explore the possibility of a 'caution and letter of apology', but an apology had already been given. At the same time, she is anxious to secure diversion from prosecution. She suggests to Jason that he write a *further* letter of apology, to show his remorse, and 'because it seems silly to have to go to court about a thing like this'. Jason agrees.

Donna then goes on to discuss with Jason and the residential social worker the role of Steven, the co-accused. Steven lives nearby. In the opinion of staff at the Children's Home he is a bad influence on their residents and has been discouraged from making further contact with them. It is felt, in relation to this offence, that Jason has been 'set up' by Steven, who is regarded as shrewder and more aware of the possible consequences.

Concluding the discussion, Donna says that she will recommend a caution and reparation, and will let Jason know the outcome.

Pre-liaison visit to Steven Rouse

Steven is on a supervision order for previous offences, and it is his social worker, Joe, from the YST, who undertakes the pre-liaison visit. Joe is worried lest, by denying guilt, Steven will be pushed up the tariff, as the police may then prosecute in order to prove his guilt. Steven comes from a large family which is well-known to the police. It seems that he has a habit of pleading not guilty, however blatant his involvement in an offence. Joe tells me that he has already talked to Steven about this offence, and that in his opinion Steven is telling the truth on this occasion.

We visit Steven and his mother at home. The house is comfortable and Mrs Rouse appears friendly. Other children are coming in and out of the room all the time. Joe talks mainly to Steven.

Joe: Are you saying that you did do this offence, or that you didn't?

Steven: I didn't. (He is quite calm and definite about this.)

Joe explains that he finds himself in a delicate position, as it would of course be quite wrong of him to suggest that Steven should say he did commit the offence when he didn't – 'and if you didn't, Steven, then of course you must say that you didn't' – but quite honestly, since the offence involved only 90p, if Steven were saying he had done it he might well only get a caution, but if he maintains that he didn't, he may end up in court . . .

Steven sticks solidly to his story, saying, 'Well, I didn't do it, and that's that.' His mother begins to talk about the injustice of it all, saying that she accepts that he has been in trouble in the past, but that this time she thinks he's innocent and he's likely to be punished for something he didn't do.

Joe: The problem is, Steven, that people may not believe your story. How do you feel about that?

Steven: Bit angry, I suppose.

Joe: Mm'hm . . . well, I have to say, Steven, that on this occasion I believe you . . . and of course I can't twist your arm to say different . . . I'll put your case forward, but you know what the police are like: it may end up in court.

He brings the interview to a close.

Second liaison meeting

This meeting is attended by a police sergeant, senior social worker, probation officer, and the two social workers responsible for the PLVs to Steven and Jason. At the start it is agreed that since Steven continues to deny the offence, his case will be dropped. The police have decided that Jason's evidence would be discounted. It is now only a question of deciding upon a disposal for Jason.

The police sergeant goes over Jason's previous offences: he has received several cautions, the last being for shoplifting in 1986.

Donna: I'd like to suggest caution and letter of apology. I don't think a PA (personal apology) is on – he can't be expected to go back again – and I don't see why the victim would want him to. (This is the first time the victim's wishes have been mentioned: this reference is used as a negotiating ploy, to support the case for a low tariff response.)

Sgt: Why don't you approach her to find out?
Donna: Yes, I could do that . . .

She no longer argues that such a meeting would be asking too much of Jason: her primary concern is to secure diversion from prosecution. She is therefore prepared to capitalise on the sergeant's apparent willingness to accept this.

Sgt: Although he's had three cautions, I'm willing to accept another with reparation . . . but it's about time he moved up the tariff because of his previous.
Donna: What about the 90p? Should he pay it back?

Senior Social Worker and Probation Officer: No, we can't get involved in that . . . and anyway, he's given her the chocolates.
Decision: Caution plus personal (i.e. face to face) apology. The reparation officer will be asked to approach the victim to find out if she would be willing to accept a visit, or letter, from Jason. Jason will be asked if he'd agree to make such reparation after he has been cautioned. It is agreed that should either party refuse, reparation will be dropped and Jason will just be cautioned.

A visit to the victim

David, who is a police sergeant and the team's reparation officer, plans to visit Mrs Marsh, the victim, one Thursday afternoon. Just before we leave, David telephones Mrs Marsh, making contact for the first time.

David: Hello my dear, is that Mrs Marsh? My name is Sergeant Moore, from Exeter Youth Support Team – nothing to worry about – I wonder if I could just pop round with a colleague of mine to have a word about the boys who took your money . . .

She agrees, apparently.

We go there straight away. A frail, elderly woman greets us at the door. David shows his identity card. We go in and sit down.

Mrs Marsh: They admitted taking it, you know . . .

David: As you may know, the boys have been identified and dealt with . . .

(It is never made quite clear that only Jason is admitting guilt and being asked to apologise.)

Mrs Marsh tells us that she found a box of chocolates, soaking wet, on her return from holiday after Christmas. She had to throw them away, but had seen the note of apology from Jason before doing so.

David: Oh, that's a shame you had to do that – but the thought was there.

He takes this as his cue to say that the police want to caution Jason for the offence and, because he was unable to meet her the first time he called, they want him to come and apologise to Mrs Marsh again.

Mrs Marsh says immediately and emphatically: 'No, no, no, I don't want them here. Not that. Nice of them to apologise, but . . .'

David accepts this without demur and suggests a letter of apology instead.

Mrs Marsh: No, no, I want *nothing*: let them keep the money and enjoy it.

(Her ambivalence is apparent here: she is half inclined to regard the boys as naughty children and half as threatening offenders with whom she wants no contact.)

David: (immediately) OK my love, I respect your decision.

He reassures her that the offenders will definitely not visit, whilst reiterating that the thought was there (thus asking her to accept the spirit of an apology).

Then they discuss how much money was taken. Mrs Marsh wonders . . . was it 18/6d? Or only 18/-? It was her newspaper money anyway.

David tells her that it was 90p and that 'in the normal way of things' he'd have liked to suggest voluntary compensation (the word 'voluntary' is used to distinguish court-ordered compensation from money paid in any other circumstances). But, he explains, the offenders live in 'a home' (only Jason does, in fact) and they don't have much of a family life, or much money.

Mrs Marsh chimes in sympathetically: 'No, no, we can't ask them for money. It's not much of a life for them.'

David tells her that he won't tell Jason that she had to throw away the chocolates because he'd be disappointed (thus reinforcing the idea of Jason's sincerity of motive). He further develops the image of Jason's remorse, saying that it was he who had wanted to give her the chocolates; nobody had prompted him (in fact, the YST hadn't done so, but his mother had, as Jason was the first to admit).

David finishes the interview with some community policing. Mrs Marsh is telling him about the various strangers who have been coming to her door recently. David reminds her to keep the chain on her door and to ask to see their ID cards. She appreciates his concern. Thanks are exchanged all round. We leave.

The interview lasted about twelve minutes. It was striking for its briskness and for David's immediate acceptance of Mrs Marsh's refusal to meet Jason.

Case Two

Richard Rowe
We follow Richard's case from his being formally cautioned for theft of twenty cigarettes to the point where he returns to the shop in order to apologise.

The caution

The Inspector invites Richard and his parents into the room and asks them to sit down. She is friendly, but firm, and talks briskly and directly to Richard, unless specifically directing comments to his parents.

Insp: I presume you know why you're here today . . . (She goes through Richard's recent offences.) And you've admitted them? Yes? Right. You're old enough to know that you could be taken to court for these offences, and your record could be held against you for life, but we're asking you instead to accept a *caution*, and provided you don't offend again, you'll hear nothing more about it. But if you do, it's citable in court. We can't go on giving you chances . . . because it would appear you've been stealing over a number of months. We want to reinforce the caution by asking you to go along to the newsagent's to make an apology. Let me explain . . . The Youth Support Team runs a reparation scheme: we ask juveniles to give an apology, in a meeting with the victim or by letter, because we believe it's a good way to reinforce a caution, to discourage you from offending again. A policeman will organise it with the newsagent and take you along to make the apology. (To the parents) How do you feel about that? Would you feel happy?

Mr and Mrs Rowe (together): Yes . . .

Mrs Rowe (to Richard): And how do you feel about it?

Richard: Don't mind . . .

Inspector: (laughing) Looks like the decision's been made for you . . . Anyway, as I said, the policeman will organise it all for you, contact the newsagent, and then he'll be in touch with you.

The Inspector asks Mr and Mrs Rowe and Richard to sign the caution forms. She escorts them from the room.

Mr and Mrs Rowe appear well satisfied with the process. As for refusing the invitation to apologise to the shopkeeper, it would take an extremely brave or foolish offender to do that in this context. It would be embarrassing for his parents and would also challenge the Inspector's authority.

Arranging the apology

The file is then passed to David, the police sergeant who acts as reparation officer. He begins, a few days later, to arrange the apology. As he explains it to me:

'We'll go to the newsagent to see if they'll accept – because if they don't, then that's that, end of story. Then if they say "yes", well, we can go round to Rowe's house, tell him "put your coat on, boy" and get it done there and then.'

The shop is a small, old-style newsagent, with boxes of loose sweets all around the till. A woman in her sixties is serving.

David: Good afternoon ma'am, my name is Sergeant Moore, and you'll be Mrs Hobbs? I wonder if I could have a quick word? Nothing to worry about.

The woman explains that she is Mrs Hobbs' mother. Mrs Hobbs has just gone home with her children. She is due back at any moment.

David asks if we might still have a word. Going through the file, he says: 'Now, you may remember those two lads who stole the cigarettes?'

'Yes,' she says immediately, 'I do.'

David begins to explain that Richard has been cautioned, at which point the daughter returns. It is explained who we are. Mrs Hobbs takes over from her mother.

'Now, Mrs Hobbs,' says David, starting again, 'the young rascals who nicked these cigarettes . . . one of them wants to make an apology to your husband . . . he's been caught and cautioned and wants to apologise.'

(Put like this, it would appear churlish to refuse.)

David: I suppose *you* could do it: it doesn't have to be your husband . . .

Mrs Hobbs agrees, rather doubtfully.

David: What we'd be doing is bringing him here, not for a telling-off, because he's had that at the police station, but for you to point out to him the folly of his ways.

(Mrs Hobbs is looking *very* uncomfortable about this.)

David takes an Aero bar from one of the shelves.

David: Say he'd nicked an Aero, it's a matter of telling him, 'we haven't just lost an Aero; it's all the inconvenience, and we have to sell more stock to make up for it' – all that sort of thing.

(The emphasis has now shifted from simply accepting an apology to providing an appropriate response.)

Mrs Hobbs suggests that her husband may be better suited to do this and asks if David could have a word with him instead. They discuss when Mr Hobbs might be available to receive the apology. It is now assumed that the idea will be acceptable to Mr Hobbs – any further contact will be about organisational details.

We leave and drive to the offender's house.

Richard himself opens the door. He appears shy and awkward. David introduces himself, telling Richard that he has nothing to worry about.

David: Now, you remember that you were cautioned the other day and agreed to make an apology? Well done for that Richard, thank you, that's a good start. I'm here to arrange it.

They discuss times when the apology might be made. David thanks Richard again for agreeing to apologise, exhorts him not to re-offend, and says he'll be in touch.

The apology

The meeting takes place one lunch-time, two and a half weeks later. David has visited Richard the previous evening in order to make sure he is prepared. Richard was worried, apparently, fearing that the shopkeeper was intending to hit him. David reassures him that there will be no violence whilst he is there – 'that's not what it's all about'. He has also visited the newsagent, Mr Hobbs, and briefed him as to what to do – that is, not to give the boy a telling-off, but to explain the problems associated with this kind of offence.

We arrive at Richard's house. He is at the window, waiting, and opens the door immediately. He looks smart and very nervous. David is friendly, ribbing him about what is to happen.

David: Just apologise to him – don't have a smirk on your face, or he'll smack you one! . . . Got your boxing gloves?

A little later.

David: Right. When we get there, I shall go in . . . and if he comes out with a shotgun and you see me running, run for it yourself . . . (Richard grins with relief: he is sure this is a joke).
What's the value of the cigarettes? £1.50? It may be – not that I'm making you, mind – that you may want to offer to pay him back for the cigarettes. In your heart of hearts, you might think that's fair. It's his loss, after all. What about the other boy? He's going to court, isn't he? Keep out of his way. He's bad news with a capital B. Now, you know what you've got to say? It's up to you if you want to pay him back, but it seems a fair thing to do. Nervous?

(There's no doubt that he is; Richard indicates as much.)

David: Good.

We reach the newsagent's. Richard is told to stand by the car, while we go in to see Mr Hobbs. He is ready and waiting, very co-operative, and anxious to do the right thing. David, friendly and relaxed, explains to him that Richard is nervous, as he is expecting to be beaten up. Mr Hobbs laughs, saying 'No, no, it'll be nothing I'll be saying . . .'

(Both participants are now geared up to giving a performance in the interests of the other.)

David ushers Richard into the shop. The apology takes place in the shop itself, with customers coming in and out and occasionally wandering past Richard and Mr Hobbs.

David: This is young Richard.

Richard stands there, hands clasped behind his back, looking anxiously at Mr Hobbs. He mumbles: 'I'm sorry . . . I could pay for the cigarettes.'

Mr Hobbs takes this as his cue: 'That's the least you could do really . . . it's not just the stealing – 2p a packet we make. The only reason you got away with it is your age. It's not just the theft, it's the repercussions . . . someone bounced a cheque on me the other day . . .'

(He goes on to describe the problems arising from the cheque offence.)

Mr Hobbs is trying to perform a public duty to the best of his ability. He manages to say why the theft was a problem to him, and also takes the opportunity to try to persuade Richard not to repeat the offence. He occasionally looks to David for reassurance, which David gives, through nods and smiles. Richard takes all this meekly.

Mr Hobbs: At least you had the guts to come and see me, though you had to take a bit of prodding. You needn't pay back the whole £1.50 at once. I don't want you just to get it off your mother and forget all about it. If you can just afford 20p a week, I'd appreciate that. Save it up yourself – it was you who smoked them. Then, if you give me the money, we'll forget all about it. Think about what I've said.

(It appears that Mr Hobbs is trying to ensure that this is a *meaningful* occasion, he is not particularly interested in getting the money back.)

Mr Hobbs says goodbye to Richard, who leaves the shop. David thanks Mr Hobbs, who replies: 'That's OK, I just hope it helps.' He appears pleased. Richard has conveyed the impression that he'll think twice before shoplifting again.

On the return journey David asks Richard if he's feeling better. He says he is. He certainly looks better.

David: That's good. Well done boy. You did a good job. I'll give you his number so that once you've saved the money you can give it him back. This will be the first and last time we meet in these circumstances . . . won't it? If you should need me about anything in future – help, advice, not just about thefts, just get in touch. I'll give you my card.

Case Three

Gary Hobday
Gary has made hoax emergency calls. He is asked to apologise to officers of the Fire and Ambulance services.

We were unable to observe the reparation officer's prior visit to Gary and his parents, or the preliminary negotiation with representatives of the two services. The reparation officer, Sergeant Moore, informs me that he has told Gary that he is to apologise, that he should call the officers 'sir', and that he is to dress smartly. He also describes his conversations with officers at the fire and ambulance stations. He has told them that Gary has been caught and that 'by way of punishment, for want of a better phrase', he is being asked to apologise.

On our way to collect Gary, David explains that he called to see him for a second time the previous evening to remind him to be ready at the appointed time, smartly dressed.

We collect Gary at 9.45 a.m. His mother, smiling and friendly, waves him off: we might almost be taking him on a school outing.

Gary is overweight, slow-thinking and placid. David is full of fatherly advice.

David: So you know what you're going to say?
Gary: (mumbling) . . . Got to apologise . . .
David: Apologise. Call him 'sir' . . . Just say 'I'm very, very sorry, *sir*. It won't happen again.' And it won't, will it?
Gary: No . . .

We arrive at the Fire Station: Gary appears anxious now.

David: How are you feeling? Nervous?
Gary: Not really . . .

David asks Gary to remain at reception while he checks with the Deputy Chief Fire Officer that all is ready. (This is part of the treatment, David tells me, 'to leave him sweating' for a few minutes.)

We introduce ourselves to the Deputy Chief. Gary is led into the room by David, directed to a seat, and introduced.

David: Now Gary, I think you've got something to say to the
              gentleman . . .
Gary: (quick and mumbled) I'm very sorry for making the
              phone calls.
Fire Officer: How many did you make?
Gary: Two.
Fire Officer: Why?
Gary: Because I wanted to get other boys into trouble.

(In response to further questions, he explains briefly about his being
bullied at school.)

The Fire Officer then makes a restrained speech, explaining the
risk to life and waste of resources caused by hoax calls.

Fire Officer: (finally) Well, you've said you're sorry and I accept your
              apology.

David ushers Gary out of the room. He thanks the officer for his
help. I ask Gary how he feels now.

Gary: A bit better. I thought he'd be much crosser, that he'd have
          a go at me.

We set off for the Ambulance Station. In the car, David talks to Gary
about the problems of bullying at school and Gary's future job
prospects (which are slight), before preparing him for the next
apology.

We are ushered into the office of the Chief Ambulance Officer.
He asks Gary to sit rather than stand, perhaps wishing to avoid any
impression of this being a dressing-down.

David: I think you have something to say to the officer, Gary.

Gary mumbles what is presumably an apology.

The Officer, apparently satisfied with Gary's effort, and rather
embarrassed, says: 'Fine, fine, I'm not here to tell you off because I
realise you will have had your ear bent like that already.' He briefly
explains the workings of the service, and then seems at a loss, finally
suggesting that Gary might like to see the control room. (This really
is like a school outing.)

We all troop in to the control room, which is full of people in
uniform, machines, and flashing lights. Gary is passed to someone
who can explain the system to him in more detail.

We hang back with the Chief Officer. After five minutes or so,

Gary is returned to us. The Chief Officer says to David: 'That should be OK, then?' (Have I performed the task required?) David thanks him; shakes hands; we leave.

Gary has had a good time. He is interested in the workings of the place, and he's probably received more attention, and concern for his well-being, than he has in weeks. He relaxes now that his apologies have been made.

In the car David chats with him, offering to send in police officers to stamp out the bullying at school. Gary doesn't take him up on this. David also encourages Gary to do more housework and to work harder at school.

We arrive home. Mrs Hobday is very appreciative. She complains about the poor police response when she'd received the hoax calls (Gary had directed the ambulances to his own address). David apologises on their behalf. They discuss the bullying, which sounds quite extreme. David reassures her that it's not her fault. He also informs her that Gary has apologised – 'so he won't be playing those tricks again'. Mrs Hobday appears to appreciate the time afforded her to talk about her problems, quite apart from David having arranged the apologies.

David leaves his card, telling Mrs Hobday that he has instructed Gary to ring him rather than get in trouble again, and he'll try to help: 'The Youth Support Team – that's what we're here for.'

They both wave goodbye to us.

Gary re-offended (attempted theft) a few weeks later: his mother immediately telephoned the Youth Support Team – which suggests that David had been successful in his attempt to portray the team as a source of help. Following this second offence Gary was placed under voluntary supervision, thus further underlining the scheme's triple responsibility for diversion, offence resolution, and the provision of a support service for children and families.

Case Four

Mark Rowlands

In this case we observed an apology for the theft of a wallet taken three months previously from the car of a teacher at the offender's school. £15 was stolen (the wallet later retrieved) and the car window smashed. The offence came on top of other transgressions, so Mark was suspended from school. In addition his father insisted that he leave home. He was therefore admitted into local authority care under a voluntary care order.

At a liaison meeting in January it was agreed that Mark be cautioned and asked to apologise to the teacher.

Mark had previously committed several thefts and burglaries. At the time of this latest offence he was attending an Induction Group run by the Youth Support Team. It was through this group that he knew Michael, the social worker who organised the apology. Michael had not previously undertaken this task which was normally the responsibility of the reparation officer, a police sergeant, although other social workers in the team had performed it in the past.

Michael has already discussed the offence and the events surrounding it with Mark. He has also visited him at the Children's Home in order to plan the apology. Mr Symes, the victim, has agreed to meet Mark.

On the morning of the scheduled apology Michael wonders whether it would be appropriate to arrange cash compensation for Mr Symes. However, he gathers from others in the Youth Support Team that Mark has so many fines and other debts outstanding that it is unlikely that he could pay, or that Mr Symes would expect him to do so. Michael has informed Mr Symes that Mark has been cautioned for the offence 'due to problems at home'.

The apology

We collect Mark from the Children's Home. He appears a young fifteen, scrawny and friendly. On the journey Michael discusses the offence and the pending apology.

Michael: I spoke to Mr Symes on the phone and told him you'd been cautioned and that you were expected to apologise to him. He said he'd be pleased to receive your apology. What are you going to say?

Mark: I'll think about that when I get there.

Michael: Does he know you're in care?

Mark: Don't think so.

Michael: You could mention that. Would it be terribly embarrassing for you to explain that what you did was because you were very unhappy at home?

Mark is non-committal.

Michael: What you said about it being chance that it was his car . . .
that would be useful . . . that it wasn't because you'd got it
in for him.

Mark: Yes, it could have been anyone's.

Michael: His insurance covered the window but he's out of pocket
by £15. Would you be prepared to make him an offer?

Mark: Yes . . . might as well.

They discuss Mark's limited resources.

Michael: So you could say to him, 'I haven't got much money at the
moment, but I could pay so much over a number of weeks.'

We arrive at the school. It is the first time that Mark has returned
since his suspension, so he is a bit tense. Michael asks him to lead the
way to Mr Symes, the games teacher. Once inside the school, Mark
acts differently, apparently very cocky, swaggering down the corri-
dors, banging out a few chords on the piano in the school hall, and
knocking on doors trying to track down Mr Symes. We find him in
the gym, playing indoor hockey. He joins us, wearing shorts and
carrying a whistle. He says 'hello' to Mark and leads us into his
office, next to the gym. It transpires that this is also a thorough-fare
leading to other rooms. There are constant comings and goings,
knocks at the door, pupils returning or requesting footballs and
hockey sticks.

Michael, Mark and I sit on the three chairs in the room. Mr Symes
leans against a filing cabinet. Michael explains that Mark has been
given a caution, which was his 'ticking off'; and that he is expected
to make an apology, face to face with the victim . . . 'This is because
in court, one would never get to hear about the effect on the victim
and we think that's wrong . . . So, Mark is here to apologise. Over
to you, Mark.'

(Mark is now looking small and anxious, in marked contrast to his
demeanour outside the room.)

Mark: (rushed and awkward) Yeh, well, it was nothing personal,
just happened to be your car – and I'm sorry.

Mr Symes thanks him clearly for the apology. Throughout the
interview he directs his remarks to Mark, not looking to Michael for
guidance or support. He also talks to Mark in a straightforward way,
without being patronising. This has the effect of giving Mark's
apology greater weight.

Eventually Michael suggests to Mark that he have a go at describing his feelings on the morning of the crime. Mark does not respond at first. The room doesn't help – two people knock on the door during his first attempt. Michael prompts him, saying 'you weren't too happy that morning, you were telling me last time . . .'

Mark at last says 'well yes, I was a bit pissed off. . .'

At this point, the door bursts open and another games teacher comes in, chattering away, and apparently attempting some form of country dancing. It finally dawns on her that we're there for a purpose and she quietens down. Mr Symes doesn't explain what's going on. She leans on a different filing cabinet and all eyes turn back to Mark. He now has four adults watching him while he is meant to be explaining that the morning he broke into Mr Symes' car he was in a bad mood because of family problems. He is unforthcoming.

Michael begins to explain for him. The woman teacher, at last, leaves the room. Mr Symes ignores all subsequent door-knockings so that from then on we are relatively undisturbed.

Michael then raises the possibility of compensation: 'Now Mark, you were saying to me something about paying Mr Symes back . . .' He asks Mr Symes how much money was stolen, first telling Mark that the car window was covered by Mr Symes' insurance. Mr Symes says he can't remember, but thinks it was £15.

(This exchange is very awkward, perhaps because Michael hasn't properly thought it through.)

Mark mutters that he's willing to pay back the money.

Michael: When you can, of course, because you're not exactly rolling in it at the moment are you, Mark?

This is confusing. The expectation of re-payment is now being toned down. However, Michael continues by asking Mark and Mr Symes how they propose to arrange for the money to be returned. Mark appears to think hard, finally saying: 'Well, it's difficult, because he's going off, isn't he?'

(Mr Symes has said that he leaves this school at the end of term.)

Michael then suggests, rather vaguely, that should Mark continue to be motivated to pay back the money, he (Michael) – or someone else from the YST – could pass on the cash to Mr Symes.

Now both parties are muddled and conversation peters out. The door-knocking is getting more frequent. Michael suggests that we think about winding the interview up. But first he asks Mr Symes whether he has any questions for Mark. He does.

Mr Symes: What did you do with the other stuff in the wallet?
Mark: Flushed it down the toilet.
Michael: Well, that was a bloody stupid thing to do, wasn't it,
    Mark . . .

Mr Symes then lists the other items lost (including photos and credit cards) and briefly indicates the problems involved in getting replacements for everything.

This comes across well, being spontaneous and direct: it almost feels as if Mr Symes is getting something out of this part of the interview – expressing his annoyance and frustration, perhaps.

Having vented his irritation, Mr Symes thanks Mark again for his apology, saying, 'I appreciate that it can't have been easy.' They shake hands. Michael thanks him. We leave.

On the way back, Michael congratulates Mark, repeating, 'It can't have been easy.' Mark seems pleased, and says he thinks Mr Symes is 'alright'.

Michael and I discuss the case afterwards. This being the first apology that he has organised, he is impressed by its power. He thinks that practice guidelines could be useful. He also begins to consider the advantage of promoting an exchange of views between victim and offender, rather than simply arranging for the delivery of an apology.

DISCUSSION

A large part of the fascination of the Exeter project lies in its inter-agency mix. We observed a continuing struggle to reconcile the different prejudices and working assumptions derived from the staff's socialisation into the culture of their parent agencies. There was a degree of convergence, no doubt, but also a strong residue of traditional police retributivism and of social workers' 'welfare' aspirations. The practice at Exeter was an amalgam of these two strands, overlain by a commitment to diversion – but a much weaker commitment than we observed at other juvenile liaison bureaux.

Where does 'reparation' fit within this heady brew? There is no doubt that the Exeter team were committed to their own version of this idea. I say 'their own version' advisedly, since the decision to invoke reparation was taken with eyes firmly fixed on the pre-prosecution tariff, of which the various forms of reparation formed the higher rungs. It was inevitable in these circumstances that the reparation organised by the YST should be almost wholly offender orientated. This was despite the fact that the team's own literature refers to reparation as a means 'to put wrong things right'. Reparation was considered only in those cases where the young person was at risk of prosecution. So, where two offenders were involved in a single offence, one of them might be asked to 'make reparation' (say, to apologise) – because he had reached the appropriate point on the tariff – whilst his co-defendant might simply be cautioned; alternatively, if his record warranted it, he might be prosecuted. There was no question, in any of this, of reparation being instituted in cases where it would be of benefit to the victim.

In fairness to the YST staff, they did not claim to be addressing victim need, or undoing the harm done by the offence. 'Reparation', as we have already indicated, was a penalty to be paid by the offender. Victims were asked to co-operate, not on the basis that reparation was likely to be of much help to them, but in order to provide a constructive alternative to the courts for these young offenders. If it did not suit the scheme's purposes in relation to *the offender*, then reparation would be ruled out altogether. For this reason it was quite common to find offenders being asked to make reparation to *one* of their victims, but not to others.

The fact that reparation formed one rung on the Youth Support Team's pre-prosecution tariff led, inevitably, to its being viewed largely in *retributive* terms – that is, as a punishment. Little thought was given, in the course of liaison meetings, to the question of what kind of reparation, if any, the offender might *wish* to make, or to what form of reparation, if any, the victim might wish to receive. In Case One (Jason Coombes), the victim had already had one letter of apology and a soggy box of chocolates; the proposal for a further apology could only be understood in terms of the team's adherence to its own pre-prosecution tariff. The *team* decided whether or not reparation was to be undertaken, and they likewise decided what form this should take. The fact that victims were not consulted, and that offenders were 'consulted' in the context of threatened prosecution, led to several inappropriate recommendations being made. This arose because the decision-makers within the YST were too distant from victim and offender – and because they were thinking purely in terms of the tariff.

As far as 'distance' is concerned, it is instructive to compare the team's decision-making in relation to reparation with that applied in relation to repeat cautions. At Exeter, the Inspector who administered the cautions chaired the liaison meeting: if she did not feel able to deliver a caution to a particular offender, that, usually, was that. There was, in this respect, a striking contrast with the decision to ask the young offender to make reparation. Of the three YST members who normally attended the liaison meetings and determined the eventual offence disposal, none had direct experience of the attempt to promote reparation: this enabled them to be somewhat blasé about the difficulties which arose from their tendency to regard an apology, say, as simply one rung on the tariff ladder. But they could not be blind to the (rather less severe) difficulty arising from the corresponding tendency to view the police caution in this light since the Inspector was there for remind them of it.

The nature of the reparation offered

'Reparation' can take many forms, some of them devoid of reparative content. It is perhaps easier to begin by indicating what reparation at Exeter is *not*. It is not material. In common with other schemes, the YST staff concluded that to try to handle money caused too many problems: offenders could rarely afford to pay significant amounts; the mediators did not relish the role of debt collector; and victims' insurance claims might be jeopardised. The offender might still be *encouraged* to make cash payment to the victim, but the YST would not get involved in or seek to monitor the transaction.

Secondly, there is very little attempt at Exeter to *mediate* between victim and offender – as, for example, in cases of physical assault, where it might be thought that the victim also bore a measure of responsibility for what had occurred. This option was rarely suggested, perhaps because it did not fit comfortably with the notion of the tariff, being hardly classifiable as a punishment. Instead, the focus was exclusively on the offender, and on possible arguments (such as difficult family circumstances, or remorseful attitude) to support diversion from prosecution. The reparation scheme, then, was asking young offenders to carry out a set task, with the help of the victim. As it was put by Mr Symes, the teacher who had his car burgled (Case Four):

> Reparation was something he (offender) had to do, rather than something I had to do . . . I mean, he was coming to me to apologise and all I had to do was sit and either accept it, or not accept it as the case might be.

This was an accurate assessment. The most common forms of reparation promoted by the Exeter scheme were written or spoken (otherwise known as 'personal') apology. Indeed it seemed to us that the term 'reparation', as employed by the Exeter scheme, was synonymous with apology. (The YST perception is different in this respect: they told us that they institute as many work-based reparations as they do apologies, but this was not the pattern in the cases which we observed.)

As far as face to face meetings were concerned, there was a greater emphasis on the offender's experience of this event than there was on the quality of the *exchange* between the parties. Compared with Coventry (for which see Chapter 4), there was much less emphasis on facilitating communication in an atmosphere of privacy and trust. Richard Rowe's apology delivered in a busy shop (Case Two) was in marked contrast to the absolute privacy which the Coventry mediators would insist upon. This is not to denigrate the performance of the reparation officer at Exeter, whom we thought was effective in carrying out the task which he had himself developed, but he was not in the business of 'healing the hurt', or of promoting exchange 'on a feeling level', to quote from one report of the South Yorkshire reparation scheme. This was even more apparent in relation to written letters of apology, such as were often proposed by the Exeter YST. Few of the young offenders brought to the YST were experienced letter writers: they generally found that the words did not flow. In that case, David, the reparation officer, had a stock of useful phrases.

None of this is to suggest that the reparation undertaken was of no value to the participants, although it could hardly be said to have been emotionally revealing. What the face to face encounters *did* offer arose from the fact that they were almost invariably meetings between an adult and a child. The benefits, it seemed to us, lay in the fact of the young offender being faced with a decent, non-punitive adult victim who, rather than displaying anger, was prepared to give time to explaining the harmful consequences of the behaviour in question. So whilst the reparation fostered in Exeter was regarded, for the most part, as a further rung on the pre-prosecution tariff, its actual execution was educative in approach. This was why victims were given a certain amount of coaching, with the reparation officer in the role of instructor. They were told that it was not their task to tell the offender off (he or she would already have received a police caution), but to receive the apology and then to explain the consequences of the offending behaviour.

We cannot judge what effect these meetings had in the longer term, if any, but it seemed to us that at the time at least they did not lack power. Case Two provides a good example. Despite the hectic nature of the entire event, it appeared to have meaning for Richard. Although David, the reparation officer, told him what to say, and how to say it, and indicated in a way which hardly brooked contradiction that he should offer to pay for the cigarettes, Richard was responsible for his actions once confronted with Mr Hobbs. He could not easily dismiss the fact of his having apologised, as he may well have done had he really felt that the apology was given under duress. David's non-punitive approach, and that of the victim, contributed to this. Both appeared genuinely concerned that Richard not behave in this way again.

In Case Three, on the other hand, it was difficult to say what effect the two apologies had on Gary. They certainly caused him some anxiety, which might have been sufficient to put him off making further hoax calls. What he seemed to derive most benefit from, however, was the attention and the fun of learning more about the fire and ambulance services. The problem of bullying, which he indicated was the reason for his offences, remained unresolved. Cases Two and Four were perhaps more typical in that Richard Rowe and Mark Rowlands were clearly impressed with their reception, whilst Mr Hobbs and Mr Symes, noting the reaction in each case, also concluded that the exercise had been worthwhile. This was despite the fact that Richard and Mark may well have felt that they had little option but to agree to meet their respective victims.

The Exeter scheme offers a striking illustration of the highly circumscribed 'voluntariness' under which offenders may agree to make reparation to victims in the shadow of criminal prosecution. This is despite the fact that the decision to caution is not made conditional upon an offender's agreement to make reparation. At the police station, when a caution is administered by an Inspector, with embarrassed parents in the background, a refusal to accede to this suggestion would be a spectacular act of defiance. The reparation officer was himself aware of this. He stressed the importance of the offender *wanting* to make reparation, but at the same time acknowledged that this option was put to them immediately after they had been cautioned – so that they would be likely to do anything, including jump off the bridge into the river Exe, if asked to do so by an authority figure. (There is also the point, which may or may not occur to a young person in these circumstances, that whilst declining to make reparation will not lead to any additional penalty for this one offence, it is unlikely to be forgotten should he or she ever be in trouble again.)

The discussions at the liaison meetings made it quite clear that team members did not regard reparation as an *option* for offenders at the cautioning stage, although that is technically the case. It was treated as an offence disposal like any other. This was also how most victims understood the position. As Mr Symes put it, in Case Four . . . 'Mark had been cautioned for the offence and part of his, I don't know, sentence if you like, was to come and apologise to me in person.' This element of pressure might be experienced by victims as well as offenders, although clearly the degree of compulsion was not nearly so great in their case. The approach to Mr and Mrs Hobbs, in Case Two, was couched in terms which made acceptance of an apology almost as non-negotiable for them as was its delivery for Richard. However, where the victim refused, as did Mrs Marsh in Case One, then the decision was accepted without demur. (From the point of view of the Exeter YST's *diversionary* objective, there is of course no need to bring pressure on victims: the decision to caution has already been taken. Pre-prosecution schemes which seek to promote reparation in order to present a stronger diversion case to an independent decision-maker may be much more inclined to bring pressure to bear on victims, as may court-based schemes which seek to promote reparation in order to mitigate sentence.) At Exeter, the only obvious pressure experienced by the victim arose from the reparation officer's presentation of the young offender in an extremely sympathetic light . . . as *wanting* to apologise, and so on. Offenders were presented as unfortunate, foolish and regretful, rather than as dangerous and malicious. No doubt this was usually the case.

For all that I have said about the element of compulsion or inducement which underlies the offender's decision to 'make reparation', I accept that some young offenders genuinely *want* to apologise because they feel ashamed of what they have done. Even where the offender was given a very strong push, as was the case with Richard Rowe, the fact of his, technically speaking, being *asked* to apologise, rather than being required to do so, may still have made a difference. It may have made it less easy for him to deny the evidence of his own regret.

The approach of the Exeter YST towards securing agreement to make reparation may be compared with that of the Coventry scheme, where there is considerable emphasis placed on ensuring that the offender makes a deliberate and explicit choice. But in Coventry, as we shall see, the offender's decision is taken in the shadow of a pending court appearance, whilst the mediator's emphasis on *choice* contributes to a rather more subtle form of coercion, linked to the offender's need to show himself in a good light to this powerful mediating figure who is urging on him the importance of making a free choice.

Conclusion

As far as 'reparation' is concerned, the Exeter YST operates a scheme, the principal motivation for which is *diversion*; whose format (as far we observed) is *apology*; and whose principal objective in practice is *offender education*. Reparation is treated as part of an offence disposal and, therefore, as a *penalty*. Even in the course of the pre-liaison visit, the social worker sought ammunition to argue for a lower tariff disposal: 'conflict resolution' was not seriously considered, or was not thought to be feasible. We saw this even in cases of assault where the offender claimed that the incident had been 'six of one and half a dozen of the other'. One may say therefore that the framework of the tariff and the need to support the case for diversion has led the Exeter scheme to operate a somewhat limited form of reparation which bypasses issues of culpability, provocation, or excuse in favour of a highly controlled, somewhat ritualised encounter between a nervous, incoherent youngster and a benevolent, slightly embarrassed adult. Typically, these exchanges reveal very little of what the parties think of their predicament, or of one another.

A second feature of the form of reparation undertaken at Exeter is that it is based entirely on offence and offender characteristics. It is assumed, perhaps because these are *juvenile* offenders, that they have little to offer victims. The victim is coached to respond non-punitively, so as to promote offender learning and attitude change. Given that reparation takes this highly circumscribed form, it might be thought that the potential for *justice* expressed in reparative terms is barely being tapped at the moment.

That is not to say, however, that the reparation promoted by the Exeter scheme is of no value. We cannot judge the effect of these encounters in the longer term, but at the time they appeared to have some impact, at least in some cases. This arose from the young offender's relief at surviving a meeting concerning which he or she had been very worried; through encountering an unexpectedly non-punitive victim (and non-punitive police sergeant); and through being told honestly, rather than in a contrived way, just what worry or other problems the offence had caused. Some victims, incidentally, also appeared to derive satisfaction from talking about their experience in this way.

Chapter 4

The Coventry Reparation Scheme

The Coventry Reparation Scheme (CRS) began life in 1985 with the aim of providing 'a service to victims, offenders, and the court'.[1] It proposed to do this by giving an opportunity for the offender 'to say sorry for the offence and to actively participate in something which may also assist the victim'; by enabling the victim 'to express feelings, obtain information and hopefully reassurance'; and by permitting the court 'to show that it cares more about victims by taking steps to put right some of the harm done to them'. It also hoped that the experience might increase offenders' sense of responsibility for their actions, thereby causing them to think twice before offending again.

The CRS is an independent project, accountable to a management committee, but it maintains close links with the West Midlands Probation Service. In its first two years the scheme was one of four experimental projects funded by the Home Office. It subsequently received additional financial support from the probation service and the Monument Trust. The staff comprises the CRS co-ordinator; two other full-time project workers; and a secretary/receptionist.

The CRS is court-based. It deals primarily with offences of burglary, theft or assault. It rarely seeks to involve itself in shoplifting offences, or offences committed against large firms or institutions where there is no one person who can be said to have suffered as a result of the offender's actions. There are other limitations on case selection which have to do with the timing of the CRS intervention and the scheme's relationship to the court. For example, it cannot act in cases where there is the possibility of a not guilty plea. Nor can it take cases where the offender is remanded in custody. Other constraints are less obvious, since they arise from local negotiation. For example, at the time of our research the CRS did not take cases where the offender was to be sentenced in the Crown Court. Nor was it the practice to seek adjournment for mediation in cases where the offender would otherwise be dealt with that very day. (In other words, the scheme normally intervened only where the case was likely to be adjourned in any event – usually so that a social enquiry report might be prepared.)

At the time of our study the CRS drew the bulk of its cases from the magistrates court. Referral to the scheme could only be made by the magistrates, but this might be 'triggered' by a solicitor, probation officer, or, more commonly, by a CRS worker. If the magistrates agreed to the suggestion they would order a twenty-eight day adjournment so that reparation might be attempted. This was often done in conjunction with a request for a social enquiry report, although the two processes were independent of one another.

THE RESEARCH

We observed all stages of mediation at Coventry, from initial referral to conclusion of the case. We were with the CRS for approximately three days per week for two and a half months, from December 1986 to February 1987. During that time thirteen cases were referred to the scheme. We followed twelve of these, involving sixteen offenders. Eleven were referred by the magistrates; the other was a 'community dispute' referred by the police. We observed five initial referrals on court premises; sixteen interviews with offenders; five interviews with victims; two joint meetings; and three court hearings at which sentence was passed.

THE CASES

I now give summarised accounts of three cases observed in the course of our time spent with the Coventry scheme.

Case One

Offender: Steven Howe (19)
Victim: Gavin Jones (19)

The offence

Howe has admitted causing Actual Bodily Harm to Jones, knocking a tooth out and giving him a cut to the mouth which required five stitches. It appears that Jones, a student, was walking in the city centre one evening with two women friends. Howe, who had been drinking, walked past him and exchanged words with the women. Howe claims that, because of this, Jones was abusive to him. Jones maintains that Howe accused him of giving him 'dirty looks'. Howe punched Jones once in the face before being dragged off by others present. Jones reported the offence and Howe made an admission. In his statement he said that he wanted to apologise for what he'd done and regretted having done it. He added, however, that 'I wouldn't change my reaction to abuse as, like everybody else, I have principles'.

The case is referred by the magistrates to the CRS. It is allocated to Rose Ruddick, co-ordinator of the scheme.

Home visit

We visit Steven Howe one weekday afternoon at 4 p.m. Steven lives at home with his father and thirteen-year-old sister. Mr Howe greets us warmly and shows us into the sitting room, where his son is waiting for us.

Steven explains that he is very tired, as a result of the long shifts he works as a croupier. Rose begins by checking that the information the scheme has about him is correct. She goes through the charge sheet, checking date-of-birth etc., and quotes from victim and offender statements.

Rose: The stories don't quite tally, but that would be expected.

Steven agrees.

Rose then tells Steven something about the CRS. She emphasises the scheme's independence, particularly from the probation service.

Rose: People in your position don't have the opportunity to sort things out and put things right with the other party. Offenders who have taken part in the scheme found it helpful to face up to things. The court provides punishment, but that often does nothing to sort out the case.

Rose then goes on to describe the potential benefits for the victim, explaining how, in criminal proceedings, the victim is left out. The scheme aims to redress the balance by giving the victim a voice.

Steven: (breaking in) I'm under no illusions. I'm willing to apologise and be punished for what I've done, but he (Jones) has made a false statement. He's made out that things are worse than what actually happened.

Rose suggests that this is just the sort of thing the two of them will wish to discuss should they meet. She goes on to read the account of the injuries given in the police file: a cut to the mouth requiring five stitches and a tooth knocked out. She suggests that these injuries are sufficiently serious to merit the charge – 'it's not just a tap we're talking about, after all'. But she also suggests that the victim may have over-reacted at the time, in panic or anger.

Rose: He may well have cooled down since. You may even find him to be quite reasonable when you meet.

Rose then asks Steven for his version of events. He tells her that he'd been with his mates from lunch-time onwards and in fact they'd already been in a bit of a fight that afternoon. When they'd all left the pub, he'd exchanged a few words with the girls who were with Jones, whereupon Jones had been abusive to him. He'd turned around and hit Jones, before the girls pulled him away.

Rose: Had the drinking had any effect, do you think?
Steven: No. Normally I only get silly, not violent. But he said I threw a chip bag at him, and I didn't.
Rose: Was he looking for trouble?
Steven: Oh no. If anyone was pushing, it was me.
Rose: Perhaps after that fight in the afternoon, you had left-over frustrations?

Steven rejects this explanation. He continues . . .

Steven: I'd want to apologise . . . and I am sorry, but I'm afraid I'd want to give him a piece of my mind. If I'd been in his position, I would never have told the police. It goes right against my principles. And even if I did, then I'd tell the truth, and not exaggerate like he did.

Rose says she accepts that from his perspective it may seem that the victim has been unfair. She goes on to suggest, however, that the victim may have a very different point of view; he may have different standards and act according to different rules.

Rose: I won't be going anywhere near the victim unless I have your permission to do so. But equally, I will respect his wishes, too. He may not want to see you. It's all about giving two adults the opportunity to sort things out. It's up to you completely . . .

Steven: I've already said I'm prepared to meet him and to apologise.

Rose: I'll be happy to approach him on that basis. It takes guts for you to do this, and I'm sure your family will be impressed. The court, of course, will take it into consideration, though whether it affects sentence or not, I couldn't tell you.

Steven then says, in a guarded and roundabout fashion, that there were reasons why he was tense that evening and ended up hitting someone. He is not prepared to divulge what these were. Rose doesn't press him. Instead, she says again: 'If you decide to go ahead, it's your meeting and his meeting. I'll be there, but it's not my job to run it.'

Rose concludes the meeting, telling Steven that she wants him to think things over and to confirm one way or another within the next few days whether he wants to take part. Should he decide to go ahead, he is to come to see her at the CRS office again before Rose makes contact with the victim.

Second interview with Steven Howe

Steven fails to keep his next appointment. Rose attempts to contact him, but it is rare that he is home and when he is, he is nearly always asleep. Rose leaves messages with his father, in the hope of arranging a further appointment. Steven finally arrives for an office interview, accompanied by his girlfriend. It soon transpires that he has been drinking and is in a volatile mood. Rose decides that there is no point in continuing the interview. Steven protests that it was fair enough to have a drink, it being his day off.

Rose: Yes, I quite appreciate that. I'm simply saying that as far as these meetings are concerned, you need to be sober. We can contact you through your father to arrange another appointment. That seems to be the best way, if that's OK by you.

Steven: Yes, yes. (He is embarrassed, it seems, that the interview is being terminated because he is the worse for wear. He leaves.)

Contacting Gavin Jones, the victim

Rose goes to some lengths to obtain the home address of Gavin Jones, via his college. She establishes that he is an engineering student who lives more than fifty miles away. Rose telephones him one evening, to tell him about the scheme and about Steven Howe's offer of apology. She also asks about his experience of the offence. It seems that he is having to have extensive and painful dental treatment to replace the tooth he lost. Rose asks him to think over whether or not he would be willing to meet Howe, and arranges to get in touch again in a few days.

Jones eventually decides that he doesn't wish to meet Howe. He feels that if Howe were the type of person to really feel sorry for what he'd done, then he'd not have committed the offence in the first place. 'I suppose I don't forgive him,' he adds.

Rose: I understand what you're saying. I mean, I think if you are really not at the point where you feel you could benefit from hearing from him, then that's as good an answer as can be. He may ask if he can write to you, because he's not that stupid that he can't appreciate the sort of position that he's put you in.

Jones tells her that Howe can write to him, but that he won't promise a reply. Rose accepts this. She asks whether Jones would like to be informed of the outcome of the court case. He says he would.

Third interview with Steven Howe

Steven arrives on time for his next appointment.

Rose: (firmly and briskly) I've spoken to Mr Jones at some length, twice. You've created a lot of problems. He has had to spend hours at the dentist because of you, having root transplants . . . (Rose describes the treatment in more detail). Mr Jones isn't based in Coventry. He is on a sandwich course, so he is in industry at the moment. He could have done without all this on top of everything else. And he had to go home to his parents looking very different from when he left – his face was in a pretty bad state, so they were none too pleased either.

Steven: I didn't intend to do anything severe to him. I mean, I'm not making excuses, but I don't go around just hitting people out of the blue. I just didn't intend the damage.

Rose: I'm not sure how much better that would make him feel, that you didn't mean to do as much damage as you did. At the end of the day, he lost a tooth and needed five stitches. Perhaps you need to take responsibility for that. The scheme's job, in part, is to get people to acknowledge responsibility for their actions, whatever they may have intended.

Steven: (shifting uncomfortably) Yes, yes, you don't have to tell me that.

Rose describes in more detail Gavin Jones's return to the family home. Steven is embarrassed and turns to me (researcher) saying awkwardly: 'I'm not really smiling.' Rose tells Steven to ignore me and continues relentlessly – still without telling him whether or not the victim has agreed to a meeting.

Rose: He has never had such an experience before. It is quite exceptional, and not something he is likely ever to forget. Having said that, you haven't completely destroyed his life . . . he sounds to be quite a sensible sort of bloke, quite together. He said that until I'd contacted him, he would never have dreamt of agreeing to see the bloke who'd done such damage to him. He thought about it very seriously – very seriously indeed. I phoned him again to find out his decision. Finally . . . he decided against a joint meeting.

(Steven visibly relaxes at this point. His voice is stronger and he sits straighter from now on. Afterwards, Rose tells me that she deliberately delayed telling him – 'for maximum benefit'.)

Steven: I thought he'd say that.
Rose: But he'll take a letter from you. You could write it now, in one of the offices here.
Steven: I'd like to think about it first. I'll do it, but I want to give it some thought.

Rose arranges a time when Steven will bring the letter to the office. She advises him to let his solicitor know what he's doing. Steven says he'll do so, adding that his solicitor had written to him reminding him of the importance of co-operating with the scheme.

Rose: I, or someone from the scheme, will be present when the case goes back to court, to present our report.

Steven does not in fact deliver his letter.

Court hearing

On the day of the hearing Rose meets Steven in the waiting area of the magistrates court. He has his letter to Jones in his hand. He is wearing jeans, and trainers without laces. He is pale and again looks utterly exhausted. He tells Rose he was unable to bring in the letter because he had flu. Rose asks his permission to photocopy the letter so that it can be shown to the magistrates. He agrees. She gives Steven her report to read, checks with his solicitor that he has a copy, and tells them she'll see them after they've read it through.

When we return, Steven is looking upset.

Steven: This isn't what I said to you! The offence
                                sounds completely unprovoked!
Rose replies, very calmly: This is what I heard and understood you to
                                say.

An exchange follows in which it is established that Steven agrees he was the first to hit out, and that the *blow* was not provoked, even if the victim might have been abusive to him. Rose advises him to tell his solicitor if he wants him to emphasise the provocative nature of what Jones said to him.

In court, the magistrates are given copies of the social enquiry report, reparation report, and Steven's letter of apology. He is fined £100 and ordered to pay £30 costs and £150 compensation. Afterwards, solicitors and court staff remark that compensation is rarely ordered by the Coventry magistrates.

Rose writes to Gavin Jones, letting him know the outcome. She encloses Steven Howe's letter of apology.

Case Two

Offender: Brian Tate (20)
Victim: Mr Hartley (in his forties)
Tate has pleaded guilty to a charge of criminal damage. He smashed a newsagent's shop-window one night when drunk. This case was initially adjourned for a social enquiry report to be prepared. A probation officer spotted it as a 'possible' for reparation. She discussed it with Tate's solicitor who took the same view and secured Tate's agreement. The solicitor approached the magistrates the next day and they referred Brian Tate to the CRS. The case is allocated to Barbara Clark, one of the project workers.

First office interview with Brian Tate

Brian Tate arrives punctually for his 2 p.m. appointment. Barbara begins by checking if he has heard from the probation service. Then she asks about the method of referral: she'd been given to understand that his solicitor had returned to court to seek a referral to the scheme because it was Tate's specific wish to make amends.

Brian: No, not really. I was reluctant at first, but my solicitor said it would be a good idea. I thought about it and decided it was. After all, Mr Hartley didn't ask for his window to be broken. The least I can do is say sorry. Obviously I feel nervous about it, but I'll do it.

Barbara explains something about the scheme: 'It's an alternative to the courts, which runs alongside them. The courts tend to leave victim and offender out of the entire process. The scheme gives them both an opportunity to meet and for the offender to put things right with the victim.'

Brian: So what do I do?
Barbara: Well, it's not for me to say. That's up to you and the victim.

(Brian looks puzzled.)

Barbara: What I can do is outline what's happened in other cases. Sometimes the victim and offender will meet and the offender has the chance to explain himself. Or there may be a letter of apology instead. Or, again, the victim may say 'no' to taking part altogether.
Brian: (rather irritably) Well, obviously all I can do is apologise and make compensation to the victim through the courts.

Barbara turns to the offence and the circumstances surrounding it. Brian tells her that it happened after he had been made redundant. He was depressed and had had a row with his parents. He'd then stormed off, borrowed money from friends and got drunk. He'd bought a curry and sat on the wall outside Hartley's newsagent shop. His friends went home. He stayed there, feeling fed-up. Then he noticed some loose bricks lying nearby. He threw one through Hartley's window. Although a couple of his mates came by and urged him to go home with them, he stayed put until the police arrived. He was duly arrested. He was allowed to leave the police station at 4 a.m.

Barbara: What did your parents think about it?

Brian: (animated) My dad said 'If you're going to commit a crime, why don't you do something properly, like rob a bank?'.

Barbara then spends some time discussing Brian's employment problems. She encourages him to apply for courses and to take advantage of the various government training schemes. Brian is dismissive, saying that in Coventry, it's hopeless. He appears at this stage to feel little remorse for having thrown the brick. He tells Barbara of his previous offences: a year ago, on returning jobless from the USA, he got drunk and put four bricks through the windows of a police transit van. His other offence was one of 'breach of the peace' – which he says was unfair, the victim being as much to blame as he was. He was fined on each occasion. The fines have yet to be paid.

Brian talks blandly, but his words convey anger and depression. He tells Barbara that his income is £14 per week, of which £10 is spoken for. He repeatedly expresses his willingness to pay compensation for the window, despite this very low income and despite having two fines outstanding. (The compensation being claimed by Mr Hartley is £650.)

Barbara suggests that the person who suffers most as a result of his offences is Brian himself. At this he again becomes animated: 'Absolutely! You keep referring to Hartley as the victim, but that's only true judicially speaking. I'm the natural victim, and anyway, it won't have caused him so much hassle. I know, because I've worked with a window-fitter. His insurers will have sent round a firm to board up the shop, and then it would get properly mended in the morning. So, if anyone's the victim, it's me – and I'm not a criminal, I'm a bleedin' idiot!'

Barbara tells him that she'll contact Hartley to see if he's willing to take part. She warns Brian that Hartley may not be willing. She stresses that she is concerned for his interests as much as Brian's. She asks Brian to think it over and get in touch with her if he is still sure he wishes to take part. Once she's contacted the victim, she warns, she wants no backing out.

Brian: (irritably) But I've made the decision. I keep telling you – I'm telling you now – I want to take part. I've got nothing else to do all day. If he's willing to meet, let's get on with it.

Barbara is still putting the brakes on. She asks Brian to describe what he'd do in the event of a meeting.

Brian: I'd apologise of course – it goes without saying.
Barbara: Have you thought about making practical amends?

(Brian looks puzzled.)

Barbara: Doing some work for the victim, say.
Brian: I can't mend his window, can I? It's already mended!
Barbara: Perhaps you could offer to do some work for the shop.
Brian: (aghast) What?! Deliver newspapers or something? I'm not a ten-year-old!

Barbara pursues this no further. She says she will now go ahead and contact the victim on the understanding that Brian is making a definite commitment to take part. He nods at this and they arrange a further appointment to discuss Mr Hartley's response. Brian leaves.

Afterwards Barbara says she feels dissatisfied as there is little evidence of genuine remorse. She feels Brian is blaming the world for his problems. She gives him credit for waiting for the police, having smashed the windows, but other than that she is not impressed.

Barbara telephones Mr Hartley the next day

Barbara: My name is Barbara Clark from Coventry Reparation Scheme . . . You've probably never heard of it? No? A lot of people haven't. Its a relatively new scheme. (She gives a brief outline of the CRS.) I understand you've had a window smashed recently. The offender has since appeared in court. I believe he waited outside the shop for the police after he'd smashed it, so it looks as if he was already showing some regret, and taking responsibility for what he'd done. I wonder if you would be willing to discuss the matter with us . . . if you could spare the time?

Barbara persuades Mr Hartley that it would be best to meet, rather than talk further on the phone. An appointment is made for the following day.

Meeting the victim

We call on Mr Hartley at his newsagent's. The shop is small and crammed full of sweets, trinkets and magazines. Mr Hartley shows us into his office. There has just been a Christmas delivery so the office is piled high with boxes. There is no room to sit down so the interview is conducted standing amongst the boxes.

Barbara outlines the role of the CRS, saying that it operates independently of the court and that it is concerned for victim and offender equally. 'The victim is normally just a shadowy figure who gets completely left out of normal court proceedings. The scheme gives the victim a chance to have a voice in court and it also provides an opportunity for the offender to take responsibility for what he's done . . . Your case was referred to the scheme because, whatever the exact reason, the offender wants to make amends, and because he has shown some regret about his actions.'

Mr Hartley: Well, I certainly want him to take responsibility for what he's done. That's why I'm claiming costs this time. Hit them in the pocket where it hurts! Then perhaps they'll learn. (He explains briefly that he's had windows broken before, but has never bothered to claim compensation.)

Barbara steers him away from the question of compensation. She encourages him to tell her more about the offence.

Mr Hartley is obviously exasperated about the whole affair. Although he's never met the offender, he's heard from others that Brian had been depressed and was wanting somewhere to sleep for the night. He had deliberately picked the newsagent's shop because of its burglar alarm, so that he could spend the night in the cells.

Mr Hartley: In my opinion he was utterly calculating and couldn't give a damn about the consequences for others. The way I heard it, he'd simply smashed the window and then just sat on the wall eating his take-away, waiting to be picked up!

Barbara listens sympathetically. She goes on to describe the offence in more detail, presenting it in a way which is more charitable to Brian. She emphasises that it was pure chance that it was Hartley's shop. The incident reflected Brian's mood, and the unhappy proximity of a pile of bricks and Hartley's plate-glass window.

Barbara: And once he'd realised what he'd done, he came to his senses sufficiently to choose to face the consequences by staying put. And he wasn't kept in the cells all night: they chucked him out at 4 a.m. and he was told to make his own way home.

Having presented the incident from Brian's point of view, Barbara goes on to sympathise with Hartley, who nods appreciatively as she talks. She remarks on how inconvenient it must have been for him to have to deal with such an incident just before Christmas, and to have had to get up in the middle of the night.

Hartley describes with some passion just how much of a problem it had been. It seems that three bricks, not one, had been thrown. They had damaged a lot of stock and destroyed an entire window display.

Mr Hartley: What really exasperates me is that I can't see any point in it! If it had been a burglary, I could have understood.

Barbara reminds him that Tate was drunk at the time.

Hartley says that he had been worried lest his shop had been chosen deliberately and that this was the start of a campaign against him. Another shop in the row had suffered repeated damage, to the point where it had been forced out of business. Now, whenever the phone goes at night, he is on tenterhooks, afraid that it will be the police ringing to tell him of a further attack. He is also annoyed at his insurance premium having been increased.

Barbara: I can well understand how fed up you must feel about it, and about the offender's failure to appreciate the consequences. I think it would really do him a power of good to have to face the music by hearing just how much trouble he's created. A very powerful way of doing this might be if you told him yourself.
Mr Hartley: If I met him face to face, I'd probably want to break him up!

Barbara lets this go. She continues to empathise with Hartley whilst seeking to present matters in the best possible light for Brian.

Barbara: And I think the offender simply has no idea what he's put you through. The only thing we can say for him is that he waited for the police despite having ample opportunity to get away.

Hartley, for the first time, appears to soften in his judgement of Brian: 'Yes, he can't be rotten through and through. He must have a good nature somewhere underneath it all, to have stayed for the police.'

Barbara agrees immediately, as if Hartley was the first to suggest this: 'Yes, that's right, and he comes from a good family. His parents were none too pleased, either.'

Barbara appears to have won Hartley round. He begins to talk sympathetically about the problem of keeping young people on the straight and narrow. He recalls how he once made his son return with him to apologise to a neighbour for some damage he'd done. He also says that he appreciates being informed in more detail about the offender and his response to the offence.

At this point Barbara suggests that she arrange for Hartley and Brian to meet: 'I think he would have an awful lot to learn from it. And he might also go off and tell his friends about the trouble caused, so that they might think twice before doing the same.'

Hartley agrees, adding that it's about time he cleared away the pile of bricks he'd left lying near the shop-window. He expresses his approval of the reparation project. A date for the meeting is agreed. We leave in high spirits.

Second meeting with Brian Tate

Brian arrives on time but he has been drinking and is in argumentative mood. He talks to Barbara in a provocative way, at one point asserting that it is in the scheme's interests for the case to go ahead, so he is doing them a favour by taking part. Some of his comments appear to be made half in jest.

Brian: I've got to meet him anyway, because it will look good in court. I know what will happen: I'll get an SER saying that I was depressed at the time; your report will say I was prepared to say sorry; they'll hear I'm on Supplementary Benefit; and with all of that, I'll get a lower fine.

After some more conversation in this vein, with Brian apparently taking delight in challenging and upsetting Barbara, Rose Ruddick, the CRS co-ordinator, phones through to suggest that Barbara terminate the interview because Brian has been drinking. Barbara does so, telling Brian that they have run out of time, and that she'll be in touch again to arrange a further meeting.

Brian accepts this, and leaves.

In fact Barbara has two subsequent meetings with Brian, one at his home and one at the CRS office, neither of which we observe. These convince Barbara that Brian has 'the right attitude'.

The joint meeting

We collect Brian Tate at 9.30 for the meeting with Mr Hartley which is scheduled for 10 a.m. Brian is still in bed, but rapidly gets dressed. He is uncharacteristically quiet on our journey to the shop.

On our arrival Mr Hartley shows us into his office. At this stage there is no eye contact between victim and offender, Mr Hartley directing his comments to Barbara. We all remain standing because of the lack of space amongst the boxes. Barbara stands well to the side of the two men, who face each other. Brian stands with his hands behind his back and head bowed, as if awaiting sentence. Mr Hartley leans against his desk, holding a receipt showing the cost of replacing the window. It is he who speaks first.

Mr Hartley: Oh I know you! You used to go to Highfield School didn't you? (This is said in a friendly manner.)
Brian: (anxiously) Yes, I did, Why? Did I do something wrong?
Mr Hartley: No, no, no. I just recognised your face, because my son went there too.

Mr Hartley appears to have thought out what he wants to say. He gives the impression of someone seeking to perform a public service. Showing Brian the receipt, he says: 'Well, young man, you've caused me an awful lot of trouble.'

He has begun to describe the problems created, when Brian, shifting from foot to foot, breaks in to deliver a speech which he too has prepared in advance: 'Something I should say straight away – I apologise for what I did. It was a childish, stupid thing to do.'

He says this clearly, if rapidly, and looks directly at Hartley as he does so.

Mr Hartley: Thank you, yes . . . Mrs Clark here has given me to understand that you were full of remorse and that your parents weren't too happy about it either. But why did you do it?

Brian explains that, being drunk, he can remember nothing of the incident until the point when the police arrived. He says, in various ways: 'I shouldn't have done it', 'I realise it's no way to carry on', 'There was no excuse'.

When Mr Hartley himself intervenes, to say much the same thing, Brian agrees with him: 'Yes, it was mindless vandalism.'

This at first leaves Mr Hartley with little to say, other than to advise Brian strongly against heavy drinking. The exchange falters, but Barbara doesn't intervene.

Mr Hartley begins to describe in rather more detail the damage that was caused: 'You made a very thorough job of it. Why did you throw *three* bricks?'

Brian: I'm afraid I can't remember throwing any.

Mr Hartley: Well, you threw three. The first apparently bounced back and could have knocked you out. That would have served you right! (said with a grin)

Brian: (earnestly) Yes, it certainly would.

Mr Hartley: What do you expect to happen to you at court?

Brian replies, rather knowledgeably, that he expects to be referred to an Alcohol Treatment Programme and either be fined or ordered to perform Community Service.

Mr Hartley advises him to pay the fine . . . 'because the courts will hammer you if you don't' (he is unaware that Brian has fines outstanding). He again warns him off alcohol: 'Too much drink is bad for you, and you need to know your limits. I just hope you'll learn from this and won't end up going through the whole palaver again.'

Brian: Oh, I've learnt my lesson alright. I'll never do it again.

Mr Hartley asks where Brian lives, but Brian is evasive. Mr Hartley suggests an estate, and Brian replies: 'You'd think from what I'd done that I live there, but I don't.'

Mr Hartley hazards another guess and Brian says: 'Yes, around there.'

Mr Hartley expresses dismay that someone from 'a good area' should commit such an offence. Then, rather unexpectedly, he asks quite vehemently: 'Why me? Why my shop out of the whole row?'

Brian replies that it was sheer chance. Mr Hartley shows relief, apparently having still been in need of that assurance. He mutters that he is glad to hear that it hadn't been done by 'a gang of youths who'd go off sniggering round the corner'.

The atmosphere lightens. The exchanges are drying up.

Mr Hartley: Well, I think I've said about as much as I can. He's already full of remorse, his parents seem to have taken him to task over it . . .

Barbara: Yes, that's right. And at least he's had the guts to come
              and face up to what he's done.
Mr Hartley: (to Brian) I hope that you've learnt your lesson now, and
              that in twenty years' time you'll look back and
              remember this as the last time you did anything so silly.
              And I hope you pass on to your friends how much
              trouble it's caused me: then perhaps they'll think twice
              before lobbing a brick through a shop-window.

On Mr Hartley's instigation, he and Brian shake hands. He leads us
out of the office. Barbara gives him a quick word of thanks and says
she'll be in touch about the court outcome. We leave.

Brian accompanies us to the car, but says he'll walk home. He
appears in good spirits, and acts gratefully and respectfully towards
Barbara. He reminds her that Mr Hartley will need to be informed
of the court outcome, and agrees to call at the CRS tomorrow in
order to discuss the meeting.

The court appearance

Brian Tate is placed on probation for six months, with a condition
that he attend Alcohol Education sessions. He is also committed to
prison for eight days for non-payment of fines. He is not fined for
this latest offence, nor ordered to pay compensation.

Having served his time, Brian calls on Barbara to ask whether he
should inform Mr Hartley of what happened in court. Barbara
undertakes to do this herself.

She later telephones Mr Hartley. He is apparently pleased with the
outcome.

Case Three

Simon Roach (19) and David Borkowski (17).
These two well-spoken young men attempted, when very drunk, to
burgle a social club frequented by Roach (and, incidentally, by
Roach's father). They were apprehended, having caused damage
estimated at £229 in breaking in. They did not get away with
anything. It was the first offence for both. The hearing is adjourned
for 28 days in order for reparation to be attempted. The case is
allocated to Rose Ruddick, the CRS co-ordinator.

First interview with the offenders

Rose: So you found us. Which is which?
Borkowski: I'm the one with the funny name.
Rose: Where's that from?
Borkowski: It's Polish.
Rose: You should have been spoken to by my colleague at
              court, who'd have checked that you're only here be-
              cause you want to be – is that right?
              (Yes)
Rose: Because that's quite important.

Rose says that she wants to describe the scheme to them again, in order to make sure that their participation is voluntary – 'it's your decision'. She tells them that the scheme is 'independent of the court, and of probation . . . it's a service to the person on the other side of the offence – we have equal responsibility to them'.

Rose then explains the relationship between the scheme and the court: 'The responsibility of the court is first to establish guilt. Then they may wish to know more, so they may order a probation report, or, in Coventry, the case can be referred to this scheme – provided it's something you want. It's an opportunity. First, it's an opportunity to say what you think about what you did – and to try to put it right in a way that *you* want to. It's an opportunity for you to say what *you* want – not what the magistrates or anyone else wants. If you didn't give a toss, you wouldn't be interested in this scheme – because the point of it is to give you an opportunity to do what you want to put it right.'

Rose makes reference to the problems experienced by victims generally – fear and uncertainty (was their house broken into by a thug with a mask?); ignorance of what will happen next; lack of acknowledgement. Then she returns to her main theme: 'It's an opportunity for you to express how you feel; you've done something that you recognise is wrong (she hasn't really established this yet); and you want to try to put matters right. (pause) Then, on the other side, we explain to the court what you've done (reparation). We have a number of interests, but it's you who starts the ball rolling. There's no point in me approaching the victim if you're not interested.'

(Rose is striving through all this to create an impression of voluntary, indeed eager participation . . . they are here of their own volition; more than that, they are taking an *initiative*.)

Rose then returns to the awkward question (in the light of the above) of the scheme's relationship to the court: 'If you show willingness, the court may possibly look at you more leniently. Has that occurred to you?'

(Yes, they agree it has.)

Rose: The court may *well* be interested; they may take account of what you've done; but they may not; they may think that other things are more important. I don't want to string you along. There's no point going through a charade – a game. You need to think through what you did and whether personally you want to put things right.

Pause. Rose looks searchingly at the two boys: 'What do you think of the idea – facing up to what you've done to someone else?'

Roach bravely enters a caveat: 'Well, it may be OK for some offences, but I shouldn't think it would work for others, like rape.'

Rose uses this less than wholly compliant response to emphasise the *victim's* interest in the process.

Borkowski: It's OK as long as the offender knows how he can make amends – but myself, though I regret it, I don't know how I can put matters right.

This is said in an honest, straightforward way.

Rose questions Borkowski further: 'Do you feel you owe them an apology?'

'Yes – I'd face up to it.'

Then Rose asks for an account of the offence. The boys give their rather pathetic account of breaking in; failing to open a cigarette machine; realising they'd set off the alarm; being challenged by a security guard; running away – straight into the arms of the police.

Rose: Was it an ordinary day? How did you spend the evening?

They'd been drinking all evening, including at a club until 2.30 a.m. They were very drunk, looking for a lift home.

Rose asks if they weren't cold at that time in the morning.

Roach: We'd had so much to drink, we couldn't feel the cold. I suggested it – it seemed like a laugh at first – then the brain got whirring – I thought it would be a good idea.

Rose: You didn't think of getting caught?

Borkowski: (ruefully) It didn't occur to us. We didn't stop to think.

(Afterwards, when he knew that the police were after them, Roach had continued running, but Borkowski had just stood and waited for the police outside the club.)

The atmosphere in the room has become very sober and reflective. Both boys appear depressed, thinking of the mess they're in. It seems they hadn't given the matter any thought at the time. They reveal, without indignation, that the police kept them at the station for eight hours.

Rose: What are your feelings now?
Borkowski: Regret – I wish I hadn't done it.
Rose: Are you *surprised* you did it?

(This strikes a chord.)

Borkowski: Very! I just couldn't have been thinking at all, because it's not something that I'd think of doing normally.

Rose then checks their home circumstances, who they live with, and what their parents know. Roach is faced with a major problem in that he hasn't told his parents of the offence. What is more, his father is a 'regular' at the club they tried to burgle. He'd prefer them not to know: 'My dad isn't exactly a gentle person – he'd tend to go a bit barmy.' His mother, apparently, isn't much better. He says of both: 'They're not very understanding.' Rose suggests to him that his parents may flare up initially, but then calm down . . . 'It's quite a weight on your shoulders at the moment.'

(Heartfelt agreement from Roach.)

Rose checks that people at the club know who Roach is – that is to say, that he's Mr Roach's son. It's beginning to look as if this 'reparation' could have major costs for him.

Rose: (to Roach)   Perhaps you and I can come back to this in a moment (she means to exclude Borkowski).
Rose: (to both)   Perhaps we can discuss what you would say . . . (she seems to be assuming that a meeting will, in fact, take place). I'd be there, but it would be your meeting, not mine. I can't decide what you want to say . . . What would you want to get across to them?
Borkowski: Like I said earlier, I don't really know.
Rose: Let me pick out a few things from what you've said already . . . that you regret it . . .

Borkowski: Yes!

Rose: That you felt you had to apologise . . . you said earlier
              that it was something that had to be done . . . I have
              to be careful here, I don't want to put words in your
              mouth . . .

(Despite the obvious orchestration, it does appear that the two boys
are shocked and dismayed at what they've done and the plight
they're now in.)

Rose repeats: 'That you regret it; that you'd been drinking; that
it wasn't pre-meditated. You feel that an apology has to be given, but
you don't feel it would be an easy thing to do by the sound of it.'

Borkowski: It's not something I could say I *want* to do. I wouldn't
              find it easy, but it's something I feel I have to do to ease
              my own conscience (this, of course, is just what Rose
              wants to hear).

Rose: (to Roach) Does this ring bells for you too?

Roach: Yes, I wish I could put the clock back, but I can't.

Rose: I want you both to think through the basic points that
              you want to get across – first, for *you*, and then, for *them*
              (victims). Secondly, you'll be putting yourself in a posi-
              tion where you can receive what *they* want to say to *you*.

Rose then explains that she doesn't yet know whether representatives of the club will want to meet. 'They may not. Or they may
prefer to just receive a letter . . .' (How does Roach feel through all
this? He obviously has grave reservations about such meeting, but
these doubts have, for the moment, been set aside by Rose.)

Rose continues: At the meeting, it has to be what *you* want to say
                   . . . Is there anything else you want to know about
                   the club? It's my job to talk to them, but I'd like
                   to hear from you on Monday, first, to confirm that
                   you still want to go through with it. Then I'll
                   speak to the club. I will also inform the court at
                   the end of the day.

Rose then asks Borkowski to leave the room in order that she may
talk to Roach about the difficulty caused by his family not knowing
of his part in the offence.

Rose: It seems you have a slight problem . . .

Roach: A *big* problem!

Roach describes his continuing quarrelling with his parents – because of his hair-cut (punk), his clothes, and so on. He left home at one stage, but then returned.

Rose: Everybody mellows – it won't always be like this . . . You're walking round with it all at the moment.

(The underlying message appears to be: 'wouldn't it be better to get it off your chest – talk to your parents – it won't be so bad in the end'. This of course is the line she must take if 'reparation' is to proceed. If Roach meets officials of the club, they'll know who he is and his father will presumably be told.)

Rose: Have you thought about telling them – getting it over with?
Roach: It just wouldn't work. It'd probably end up with me being chucked out. He threatened to do that before.
Rose: Would it help if he found out you're trying to put things right?
Roach: The thing that would stick in his mind is it's the club where he goes.
Rose: It's your decision – if you want *me* to explain to them what you're doing – if that would water it down a bit – if you feel I could help, let me know. You've got to think how to get your apology across: (a) if your parents don't know; and (b) if they do know (still proceeding on the basis that Roach is definitely going to apologise).
Rose: Is your dad well known down there?
Roach: Yes.
Rose: Could we even bring him in on the apology? I don't want to pressurise you too much, but it's only right that I point these things out to you . . . Get back to me next week. It's something you've got to deal with one way or the other.

Rose is away on Monday, but decides she wants to talk to Roach herself. She establishes when his father will be at the pub (2–3 p.m.). She'll ring him then.

Roach suggests that Rose find out the committee's reaction first: 'If they're not willing to go ahead with it, that would be a lot easier on me . . . I'm willing to do anything to apologise, to get things straight, as long as it doesn't cause a problem with my parents.'

Rose: I'll give you a ring next week, so I can be clear where you're at. OK? Good. We've got there.

The interview ends.

Subsequently Roach rings Rose and tells her that he does not wish to meet the club officials. He feels that the risks in relation to his father are too great. (Rose has several further discussions with Roach, but these focus on his relationship with his father rather than the possible 'reparation'.)

Rose intends to proceed with Borkowski in any event. She contacts the committee of the social club who decide that it would be too much to expect Borkowski to face them all, so it is agreed that he meet the secretary, Mrs Barton, to hand over a letter of apology. Borkowski duly does this.

Roach finally writes direct to the club secretary, apologising for what he'd done. He signs the letter with his Christian name (only), in the hope that the club will not discover his true identity. He tells Rose this on the day of the court hearing. Rose rings the secretary for confirmation.

The hearing

Rose submits reports on the two boys and also tells the magistrates of the letter which Roach has sent. Roach and Borkowski are conditionally discharged for twelve months. They are each ordered to pay £114.87 in compensation.

Notice of the compensation orders was sent to the social club. At that point, since the offenders' names were given, Simon Roach was revealed to the committee as one of the burglars. He was subsequently banned from the club, but the committee respected his wishes and did not inform Mr Roach of the ban.

DISCUSSION

The Coventry scheme aims to 'provide a service for victims, offenders and the courts'. In practice, however, its role is quite restricted. At the time of our observation the CRS drew its cases entirely from the magistrates court, relying upon magistrates to make a specific request that mediation between victim and offender be attempted. This method of gathering cases was said to give the scheme 'a high profile' within the court. But it seemed to us that the CRS did not have high *status* – rather the reverse, the supplicatory position in which it was placed being one clear indication of this. The scheme was accepted in the court, but it was treated with condescension by magistrates and solicitors. It was not well integrated, being regarded as occasionally useful, but essentially marginal. Also, the hit and miss referral system was time-consuming and quixotic. It was time-consuming because CRS staff often spent whole mornings at court failing to pick up any new cases, and perhaps missing cases because they happened at the time to be in the wrong building, or because a particular defence solicitor was unsympathetic or ill-informed about the scheme. It was quixotic in the sense that the scheme wished offenders to *volunteer* to take part whilst at the same time it wanted to give magistrates a sense that they 'owned' the scheme i.e. that it was a resource for their use. This latter aspiration was at odds with the way in which the scheme presented itself to offenders – that is, as operating independently of the court.

Gaining the offender's agreement to take part: manipulation, coercion, or freedom of choice

In a few of the cases which we observed the offenders had indicated a wish to apologise very early in the proceedings (even at time of arrest), before knowing that a scheme existed which would help them to do this. But in the majority of cases the mediators found it necessary to explain the mediation and reparation concepts at some length – even, one might say, to 'sell' these ideas to the offender. The 'selling' metaphor is unlikely to appeal to the mediators, but there were occasions when we were struck by the skilful 'selling' techniques which we saw employed. That is to say, the mediator did not confine herself to persuasion by reasoning, but resorted, at times, to forms of manipulation which one might associate with salesmen or evangelists.

One example of such manipulation was the repeated claim that participation in the scheme was voluntary – 'it must be completely your decision' . . . 'it's your choice' – whilst at the same time bringing pressure to bear on the offender to take part. Participation was equated with 'facing up to' what had been done, or 'having the guts' to take part. In other words, refusal to meet the victim was stigmatised as an act of moral cowardice. One might also regard as manipulative the *presumption* that a meeting with the victim would, in the end, take place. This again was at odds with the language (with frequent references to 'making sure' and 'knowing what you're in for'). Thirdly, we noted that the mediator might refuse to 'hear' an offender's decision not to take part. If participation is to be voluntary, then when an offender says 'no' (as many do), he ought to be listened to. As it was, we noted that the mediator might *continue* to refer to a prospective meeting with the victim, as if this were still on the agenda. To continue to advocate participation in these circumstances is as manipulative (although not as crude) as planting a foot in the door. In the case of Simon Roach the mediator encountered considerable, well-founded resistance, but she nevertheless concluded her interview with the words 'Good. We've got there'. This implied, not that Roach had agreed to apologise, since he clearly hadn't, but that a difficulty had been overcome and some sort of consensus reached. To the researcher this did not appear to be the case. The dominant impression was that of moral pressure couched in the language of self-determination.

Serious moral purpose

Having expressed these reservations, I should make it clear that I am in no doubt about the serious moral purpose of the Coventry mediators. They believed that offenders ought to face the consequences of their actions. So, in preparing the offender for a meeting with the victim, the mediators were both rehearsing the offender and seeking to instil a greater sense of responsibility (and to the extent that the offender's action was deemed to be blameworthy, they were seeking to induce remorse). The assumptions were that most offenders would not have thought about these matters before; they would not have attempted to place themselves in their victim's shoes; and they might, initially, be reluctant to give serious thought to making amends, being too bound up with their own predicament.

In pursuing this educative role the Coventry mediators deliberately asked more of the offender than was strictly necessary in order to arrange a meeting with the victim. They developed a pattern of repeated preliminary interviews, often going over the same ground – 'are you sure?' . . . 'have you thought about it?' . . . 'tell me again what happened'. The message was driven home that the offence was serious – and that the decision to meet the victim was also serious, calling for a major commitment and incurring a fresh responsibility. So, although I have talked about 'selling', once the offender had given his consent, there was generally no rush to complete the process. If the offender's attitude was deemed to be inappropriate at any of these meetings – say, he turned up drunk – he might be sent away and required to think again. (I suspect, in fact, that the scheme would have been very reluctant to 'lose' a case at this stage, but they could feel fairly secure given that they were operating within the framework of an adjourned court hearing.) In these circumstances the mediators might deliberately heighten the offender's anxiety, carefully pacing their intervention in order to maximise stress. There were several references to causing the offender to 'sweat it out', sending him away to think over the prospective meeting or deliberately allowing a few days to elapse before arranging this. Likewise, if the victim had decided against a meeting, this information might not be conveyed to the offender immediately, so that he would have a little more time to reflect on his actions whilst still in the receptive frame of mind induced by the prospect of this encounter.

The problem of impure motives, or offender inducement

The Coventry mediators' attempts to raise anxiety in the offender, or to promote reflection, were made in order to combat the obvious element of inducement present in these cases. The mediators acknowledged that offenders were likely to agree to make reparation, in large part, because they hoped that in doing so they would receive a less severe sentence from the court. Of course no promises were made and the likelihood of a reduced court penalty might be played down, but the underlying message remained that the offender had nothing to lose and, quite possibly, something to gain.

As far as the mediators were concerned, the fact of offender inducement was not thought to be an insuperable problem. Their view seemed to be that, once the offender had agreed to take part, the experience of mediation and reparation was sufficiently testing not to permit him to sustain a cynical 'going through the motions' attitude. In other words, the process was thought sufficiently powerful to promote attitude change no matter what the initial motivation. We observed several cases in which there appeared to be some basis for this view.

Staging and priming

The Coventry mediators referred to their 'providing an opportunity' for victim and offender to meet, in order that they might 'sort things out'. The participants might be told: 'It's your meeting.' But to the extent that this is taken to imply participant *control* the mediators' practice was at odds with their rhetoric and, indeed, with general principles of mediatory intervention as advanced by, for example, Roberts (1983). These mediators were not unobtrusive; nor were they neutral 'facilitators'. Their style of intervention reflected the fact that these discussions took place in the context of criminal proceedings. Before any meeting with the victim, offenders were put through quite a demanding programme. The first stage of this might be termed 'victim empathy' since it involved discussion of the possible consequences of the offending behaviour for those on the receiving end. The second stage was 'meeting rehearsal', with the offender being asked to think what he wanted to convey to the victim and how he proposed to say it. Offenders were asked to put themselves in the place of the victim – 'how would you like it if . . .' – the implication being that, in these circumstances, we would all feel the same. But offenders were *also* reminded that different people view the world in different ways – for example, that a routine fist-fight might be perceived by the other party as an unprovoked assault.

What we observed therefore was the offender being 'worked on' to the point where he or she was deemed ready to meet the victim. This suggested either that the mediators had little confidence that a meeting would in fact take place (and in many cases the victim did indeed prove unwilling) or that they had little confidence that such a meeting would, in itself, serve to revise the offender's attitude. Whatever the explanation, considerable energy was devoted to ensuring that the offender came to that meeting well tenderised and so oven-ready for remorse.

It can be seen therefore that the Coventry approach involved an extremely 'active' (or controlling) form of mediation. Their practice was at odds with the view that exposure to victim anger and distress are highly effective in challenging offender rationalisation and excuse, while remonstration or exhortation by criminal justice personnel are comparatively ineffective (Walster et al, 1973; Launay 1987). The Coventry mediators might respond to this by saying that the authority and status which they enjoyed should not be equated with that of judges, magistrates, or probation officers (this may be why they placed such emphasis on their 'independence'). They might also argue (a stronger point, in my view) that these discussions with the offender took place in the shadow of a pending meeting with the victim, so that it was the anticipation of this encounter which put the offender in a receptive frame of mind.

Mediators in other contexts (such as divorce disputes) vary in the amount of preparatory work which they undertake with the parties separately, prior to a joint meeting. At some centres there are *no* preliminary meetings with the parties on their own – save perhaps for a brief chat with each at the beginning of the session (Davis and Roberts 1988). It is necessary, of course, that both sides feel physically protected; that they have confidence in the mediators' even-handedness; and that they know that they will be given space to make their statements. But this may be established through the mediators' conduct of the face to face meeting rather than through rehearsal of any kind. At Coventry, however, it seemed to be the mediators' view that the parties (especially the offender) needed to be prepared or else they would not know what to say. Now this *may* be correct, in some instances. If it *is* correct, it brings into question the existence of a quarrel, or indeed any sense of grievance. This is because people who are aggrieved, or in dispute, generally know what they want to say to one another. If, on the other hand, the parties are being invited to engage in a process which they do not understand, with purposes which are not *their* purposes, then they may well be at a loss as to what to say and need some coaching. I would suggest that, where there is an issue, coaching is redundant; and where there is *no* issue, no amount of coaching will lift the meeting out of the realm of embarrassed, forced politeness, with victim and offender each seeking to conform to the mediator's expectations of how they should conduct themselves.

The Coventry evidence is consistent with the minimalist view of the mediator's role argued by Roberts (1983). This is despite the fact that the CRS attempted to do something very different. The same mediator could preside over very different types of exchange – strained and artificial, or natural and heartfelt. In other words, it was the parties who mattered, not the mediator. Did they or did they not have something they wanted to say to one another? One might have thought that it was the mediator's task to keep the exchange within bounds, rather than to promote it.

I should acknowledge, of course, that the Coventry mediators have thought about these matters and that they have concluded that extensive preparation (mainly of the offender) is necessary and worthwhile. They believe that were they not to do this both sides would be ill at ease in an encounter which, for them, is without precedent. As a result of this lack of practice (and possibly a lack of verbal fluency) the exchange might be ritualised and perfunctory. Nevertheless, it is difficult to imagine the parties finding themselves with nothing to say if the meeting was one which they themselves had sought. Being embarrassed and tongue-tied is a condition associated with the giving of performances. This in turn suggests that victim and offender were attending under pressure, or inducement, and were seeking to follow a script prepared by others.

There are, it is true, a number of caveats which might be entered at this point. First, as already indicated, the mediators cannot be sure that a meeting with the victim will take place. Since the offender's experience of reparation may be limited to these preliminary discussions, the Coventry mediators are determined to make the most of their opportunity, using the prospect of an encounter with the victim as a stimulus. Secondly, I should acknowledge that there are circumstances when a person might want to say something (say, to apologise) but find it difficult to do so. It probably doesn't matter very much since appropriate attitude can be conveyed in a variety of ways, but this is one possible justification for rehearsal. Thirdly, and probably a stronger consideration from the mediators' point of view, is the feeling that victims, having agreed to a meeting, are entitled to a decent apology. If so, this is probably born of public relations considerations: it reflects a rather limited conception of reparative justice. After all, what victims are entitled to is *reparation*: an apology may or may not contribute significantly towards this.

It seemed to us that the emphasis on offender preparation revealed a lack of confidence in the offender – a fear that he or she would behave inappropriately – and also a lack of confidence in the victim's ability to deal with this. The CRS is interested in promoting *a certain kind* of exchange – one that will be of benefit to both parties. What is 'of benefit' is defined by the mediators. This does not require the mediators to exercise much control over the exchanges once victim and offender are brought together. The work has all been done beforehand – not least, in controlling the exchange of information. Before the parties are brought together the mediators act as a conduit of information – and we find, in fact, that much is omitted. As far as the victim is concerned, the mediators don't want to add insult to injury, so hurtful information may be filtered out. Case One, the assault by Steven Howe on Gavin Jones, was one in which the mediator was highly selective when it came to passing information back and forth. She all the time strove to identify and reinforce elements of consensus, selecting those statements which would convey acceptance of culpability, or acknowledgement of an alternative perspective.

Through all this, the Coventry mediators (the co-ordinator especially) were markedly unwilling to collude with offenders, or to let them off the hook in any way. If the offender was disposed to make excuses, or to down-play what had occurred, Rose Ruddick would listen politely, but she would return time after time to the suffering of the victim, leaving the offender in no doubt of the trouble he'd caused. She was often invited to go along with offenders' self-justificatory accounts, or to accept their portraying what had occurred as little more than a prank, but she would have none of it. She was certainly not interested in giving the offender an easy ride. Our impression was that offenders respected Mrs Ruddick for her firmness and for her willingness to convey unpalatable messages. She was not afraid to focus on the offence – and if there were difficult, unpalatable messages to be conveyed, then she conveyed them, straight from the shoulder. All this was done without rejection or insult, leaving offenders in no doubt that, ultimately, she was concerned for their welfare.

One might conclude, therefore, that Rose Ruddick's approach to mediation reflects her probation background and skills. She was concerned, above all, to make offenders face up to what they had done. She was not prepared to rely on the victim to do this and she preferred not to risk the offender meeting the victim without his having assumed the right attitude *in advance*. It might be argued that in adopting this approach Mrs Ruddick was protecting the victim. But she also took upon herself the task of promoting offender education and attitude change. Lacking confidence in the power of the victim/offender encounter as a means of promoting the kind of learning which she had in mind, she was disposed to rely, instead, on her own confrontational and therapeutic skills.

The intensive preparatory work with offenders also reflected the Coventry scheme's relationship to the criminal court. They were referred *offenders* – in other words, people whose status had already been defined. Questions such as 'how serious?', 'how responsible?', 'whose fault was it?' appeared already to have been resolved. This might explain why the bulk of the mediators' preliminary work was with offenders, rather than with victims. But the question remains as to why this preliminary work was necessary at all. I can see that the mediators may be reluctant to expose victims to unremorseful offenders, but apart from that the series of preparatory meetings could only be understood in terms of the CRS workers' limited faith in the victim/offender encounter as a means of achieving their principal objective, namely, offender learning and attitude change.

Working with victims

The Coventry mediators wanted offenders to meet their victims in order to induce a sense of remorse; but in proposing such a meeting to victims they often suggested that the offender was *already* remorseful, 'taking responsibility for his actions', and so on. The thrust of the message to victims appeared to be: 'a sincere apology is on offer – why not accept it?' This would both 'serve the offender right' (that is, the action would be painful for him to perform) *and* it would 'do him good' to have to listen to the victim's account of the suffering that had been incurred (that is, he would learn from it). So victims were offered a role in both *punishing* and *reforming* the offender, whilst being invited to show sufficient good grace to accept an apology.

Various (often rather shaky) evidence was adduced in support of the contention that the offender was already remorseful. For example, it was said that an offender's willingness to meet the victim was itself evidence of contrition, or of a willingness to take responsibility. The offender was presented as *keen* to apologise, and as demonstrating *courage* in so doing. In Case Two, the mediator, Barbara, informed the victim, Mr Hartley, that 'your case was referred to the scheme because, whatever the exact reason, the offender wants to make amends and because he has shown some regret about his actions'. In fact, Brian Tate had shown a mixture of belligerence and self-pity. The only evidence which Barbara can offer in support of her contention that Brian showed appropriate attitude was that of his behaviour immediately after he had smashed Hartley's window display: 'once he'd realised what he'd done, he came to his senses sufficiently to choose to face the consequences by staying put.' Given Brian's drunken state, it is by no means clear that he was 'choosing to face the consequences': he might equally well have been contemplating the mysteries of the universe; or digesting his curry.

This case was unusual in that the victim was approached before the mediator had any convincing evidence of offender contrition, but in general the emphasis on *achieved* remorse was understandable given the mediators' wish to secure victim agreement to a meeting, although in the case of Brian Tate it might be regarded as manipulative and therefore another example of the 'selling' techniques to which I referred earlier. (There were other cases, such as that involving Roach and Borkowski, in which portrayal of the offenders as remorseful would have been entirely justified.) The emphasis on achieved remorse was also consistent with the mediators' reliance on their *own* ability to promote offender attitude change. Rose Ruddick, especially, devoted considerable energy and skill to the task of encouraging an offender to re-think. If she were successful, it would be correct to portray the offender as already remorseful. The meeting with the victim might then be designed to achieve *other purposes*, such as: (a) reassuring the victim; and (b) completing the reparation package in the hope that this would be accepted as mitigatory by the court.

Although the CRS focused primarily on the offender, the mediators were genuinely concerned that the process offer something to victims. So they gave victims a chance to go over their experience and to express anger or hurt; and they conveyed information about the offender and about progress in the case. The careful editing that took place, particularly with regard to offender attitude, can, to some extent, be seen as a reflection of the mediators' wish not to upset victims unnecessarily. This may have been why Rose, in Case One, omitted to tell Gavin Jones that Steven Howe thought that he (Jones) had had no business going to the police and that he considered Jones's version of events to be exaggerated. Cases such as this, in which the victim declined to meet the offender, were the ones in which the mediator's tendency to take responsibility upon herself was most marked.

Whilst the CRS staff wanted the experience of mediation to be a positive one for victims, this was not their principal concern and they were quite prepared to arrange a face to face meeting in circumstances where the victim was not by any stretch of the imagination *seeking* an encounter with the offender. This concentration on offender interests was inevitable given the scheme's close relationship with the court. Since the court is exclusively offender orientated, with victim interests considered only as an abstraction, the CRS, which obtained its cases *from* the court and reported *to* the court, was almost bound to focus on the offender. This was reflected in the scheme's starting point – repeated interviews with the offender to establish appropriate attitude, held before the victim was even asked whether he or she was interested in 'reparation'. This could be seen as a way of protecting victims, but it also suggests that the CRS was principally concerned with the *offender's* experience of mediation and reparation.

Impact on the court

Although the Coventry mediators did not give offenders an easy ride, the report which they prepared for the court was invariably designed to mitigate. Even in cases where the offender had not co-operated with the scheme at all, the phrasing was carefully uninformative – and to that extent protective of the offender's position. Given that it was the scheme's intention to mitigate on behalf of the offender, what effect did it actually have? Our research method did not enable us to study a large number of cases, but such evidence as we have suggests that the impact of reparation on the sentence of the court is wholly uncertain. For example, we observed the case of one young offender who had committed several minor (albeit irritating and potentially costly) acts of vandalism. He had had a cuff round the ear at the time and he had also experienced several meetings with the mediator and one encounter with a victim, the latter occasioning him considerable anxiety. In the end this young man, who worked on a YTS scheme and whose victims were insured, was ordered to pay £260 compensation. We have to face the possibility that the mediation (and subsequent report) in this case persuaded the magistrates to be *more* severe than they would otherwise have been, because victim loss had been highlighted. Compare what happened to another offender whose case we observed: he had committed several thefts; he did not co-operate with the scheme in any way; he was older; the offences were more serious; and yet the total financial penalty in his case was £55.

Reparation was 'sold' to the offender, in part, on the basis that participation might secure a lighter sentence from the court. The mediators made no promises, but they nevertheless conveyed the impression that, were the offender to place a bet on it, the odds would be in his favour. (It was evident from the advice they gave their clients that some defence solicitors thought the same way.) This presents a paradox. The mediators did not make a great deal of the mitigatory potential of 'reparation', but it was nevertheless an important selling point because offenders were only too well aware of the potential benefit to themselves (in other words, it did not need to be sold *hard* in order to be effective). This impression management, as I might term it, was barely justified by the wholly unpredictable impact of reparation on the sentence of the court.

To counterbalance this possibility of 'double punishment' in circumstances where reparation failed to mitigate, it seemed to us that the CRS offered a more worthwhile experience for offenders than they were likely to receive at the hands of the court. They were asked to reflect on their actions; and they were treated with evident concern. They were asked to 'accept responsibility' for their future behaviour – not simply to 'accept responsibility' in the sense of 'take your punishment'. It did not seem to us that they were being reinforced in a criminal identity.

Conclusion

It is difficult to present a clinical, dispassionate account of the Coventry Reparation Scheme because, at the time of our study, this was dominated by the vision and personality of its co-ordinator. The Coventry model of mediation and reparation was her model. At the same time one can see that it is a model which has its roots in the values, priorities, and working practices of the probation service. The aspect which, it seemed to us, was unlikely to be replicated within other reparation schemes was Rose Ruddick's strength of moral purpose, coupled with her ability to slide over a number of awkward contradictions arising from the scheme's relationship to the court. To observe the other mediators attempt to transmit the same messages was to gain a better appreciation of the difficulty of the task which Mrs Ruddick had set herself and her colleagues, whilst at the same time forcing one to acknowledge the moral strength which she as a worker managed to convey. In anyone else's hands the obvious element of offender inducement would have severely undermined the other messages being conveyed – that it's *your* choice; you've got to *want* to do it; it takes *guts* to do it – and so on. But in Rose Ruddick's hands these various elements were seamlessly combined. In the end, whatever the reservations which one might have about the *coherence* of the message, offenders were subjected to a very testing review of their attitude and motivation. It was our impression that the process was much more demanding than simply being required to attend court.

It was the strength – and possibly the justification – of Rose Ruddick's method that the process *was* demanding of offenders. It could so easily have been ritualised, perfunctory and 'symbolic' . . . after all, this is what 'reparation' conducted at the margins of our criminal justice system is designed to be. The CRS, in common with most reparation schemes, was a hybrid. This was reflected in the unsatisfactory referral process and in the lack of clarity concerning such key issues as mediator authority and offender motivation. Rose Ruddick's particular skill lay in overcoming this latter difficulty, at least to the extent that she denied offenders the right to be cynical. She had also developed what might be regarded as a new and vibrant model of probation practice.

NOTE

1 This, and subsequent references, are taken from the Coventry Reparation Scheme Report for 23.9.85–22.9.86.

Chapter 5

The Totton Reparation Scheme

Totton is a relatively prosperous outlying district of Southampton, with its own magistrates court and probation office. The victim/offender mediation scheme has been in existence since July 1985, having evolved from a working party set up by the Hampshire Probation Service. The scheme still operates under the 'probation' umbrella, although at the time of our study the resources committed to it by the Hampshire service were minimal. Immediate responsibility for the project lies with a probation officer based at the Totton office, but the scheme is in fact heavily dependent upon four or five accredited volunteers. They undertake most of the mediation, acting in pairs, although the supervising probation officer also does some. The fact that most of the work is undertaken by volunteers, whilst the supervisor is a busy probation officer with many other responsibilities, has inevitably restricted the scope of the scheme.

The scheme operates at the *pre-hearing* stage. The supervising probation officer is granted access to charges and summonses which are to be heard at the Totton magistrates court (either adult or juvenile) over the next few weeks. At this stage it is often unclear how the person charged intends to plead, or whether there will be an adjournment for some other reason. If the case is deemed suitable, and if it is felt that there are the resources available to take it on, it will be allocated to two members of the group. They will make preliminary enquiries of the offender, and then, if 'mediation' appears a possibility, they will contact the victim. So, unlike Exeter, this is not a diversion scheme; and unlike Coventry, it does not operate on adjournment. The Totton scheme in fact operates a much simpler model, although it has to be said that uncertainty as to plea is a major handicap for any court-based scheme, as is the comparatively short period (three weeks or less) in which the mediators have to contact both parties and arrange a joint meeting.

As is evident from the above, the Totton magistrates and court clerk are content that victims and offender be contacted without securing the court's agreement in each case. That said, there appears to have developed an understanding that the scheme will operate very much at the lower end of the tariff. Serious assaults, for example, are ruled out. To some extent this is a matter of timing: more serious cases do not lend themselves to intervention at the pre-hearing stage. This is partly because the future legal conduct of the case may be uncertain, with the possibility of a not guilty plea; and partly because there is insufficient time to explore the consequences of more serious offending in any depth. Even amongst those cases in which reparation is deemed to be feasible, the majority are abandoned before reaching the point of a victim/offender meeting. This may be because victim or offender do not keep appointments, or decline to participate, or because the offender's attitude leads the mediators to conclude that he is unlikely to benefit from the scheme.

The supervising probation officer and the volunteers are all concerned lest the offender's decision to offer 'reparation' be too heavily influenced by the anticipated benefits (a lesser sentence) when the case comes to court. They will therefore attempt, in the course of a preliminary interview, to test the offender's motivation. On the whole they believe that the option not to participate is a real one and the element of coercion or inducement less than in those schemes where mediation is attempted on adjournment. Perhaps inevitably, however, there is an element of 'fudging' in this area, with the volunteers' 1986 report claiming that theirs was 'essentially a personalised scheme; but one which should act as a supplement to the court process'. Certainly it is made clear to the offender that if he engages in the process a written report will be presented to the magistrates. Unlike Coventry, where the magistrates will expect a report in all cases adjourned for reparation, the Totton scheme does not submit a report in cases where the offender declines to meet the victim.

It is worth drawing attention at this stage to one other feature of the Totton scheme, this being the mediators' habit of not fully explaining the purpose of their visit in the preliminary letter sent to the parties. In fact it is not stated that the letter emanates from a reparation scheme. Sometimes, indeed, it is thought better to call on the off-chance,

without any preliminary letter having been sent. The opaque preliminary letter (or the lack of any written notice) is justified on the basis
that it is difficult to explain concepts like mediation and reparation
in a letter. So the mediators prefer to do their explaining face to face.
As researchers and door-to-door salesmen are also aware, this makes
it less likely that the caller will be turned away.

THE LOW LEVEL OF ACTIVITY

According to the Totton scheme's 1985/6 annual report, the twelve
months to July 1986 saw twelve cases reach the point of a face to face
meeting between victim and offender. Then there was a hiatus, with
the departure of the supervising probation officer, plus some confusion and uncertainty about the referral system, so that few cases
were considered for mediation in the six months from July to
December 1986, and none in that time, as far as we are aware, led to
a meeting between victim and offender. This did not mean that there
was *no* activity over this period. In fact the pattern was not untypical
of embryonic ventures which are dependent on volunteer effort: the
volunteers continued to meet and to derive evident satisfaction from
their identification with the scheme; the meetings of the Steering
Group continued to their normal schedule; but the core activity
which would have given meaning to these various gatherings appeared, for the time being at least, to have been abandoned.

There were several reasons for this low level of activity, one being
the introduction of the Crown Prosecution Service in October 1986.
This led, for reasons which it would take a separate research study
fully to unravel, to a breakdown in the system whereby the police
informed the scheme of pending court appearances. It took months
for this to be sorted out. The reason why it took so long to resolve
this administrative problem, and the reason why, at the time of our
study, the Totton scheme took on comparatively few cases, was to be
found in its organisation and resourcing. The whole enterprise was
run on the proverbial shoe-string. The supervising probation officer
was expected to carry this responsibility in addition to a full caseload,
whilst some of the volunteers also had other probation tasks. This
was in stark contrast to the Coventry scheme, with its four full-time
staff. It is important to recognise, however, that it is Coventry which
provides the exception: the level of activity which we encountered
at Totton was far more typical of reparation schemes in England and
Wales.

THE CASES

I now present summaries of four cases observed at Totton between January and April 1987. I include *all* the cases observed which got as far as a face to face meeting between victim and offender, and one which did not.

Case One

Steven Pearce (15)
Steven is charged with criminal damage: throwing stones through the windows of a school. The cost of repair was £40.

The case is allocated to Carol (supervising probation officer) and June (volunteer). They have written to Steven and his mother, giving a time when they will call. Their letter refers to the pending court appearance but does not mention the reparation scheme.

20/1/87. 4 p.m. We arrive. Mrs Pearce is distracted and upset. Steven hasn't returned from school. He knew about the appointment with Carol and June. Mrs Pearce can't do anything with him. She separated from her husband last summer. He now lives on the other side of Southampton, but still sees Steven occasionally.

Mrs Pearce says she is very worried about Steven. She'd been wanting to ask – is there anyone from whom she can get help in dealing with him? Carol and June are non-committal in response to this; they're here to focus on the offence and possible mediation. Everyone is hamstrung by the boy's absence.

Carol and June introduce the subject of reparation. They explain that they would like to arrange a meeting between Steven and the headmaster of the school. Mrs Pearce thinks this would be a good idea. Carol and June are careful not to make much of the fact that Steven could do himself a favour with the court if he meets a representative of the school in order to apologise – he has to *want* to do it, they say. But Mrs Pearce is alive to the fact that this would look good in the eyes of the court. She is very upset that Steven hasn't shown up; this is symptomatic of his general behaviour. Mrs Pearce cuts a rather sorry figure – distracted and ineffectual. At one point she orders the dog out of the room: the dog ignores her.

Carol asks Mrs Pearce to telephone the probation office should Steven decide that he would like to meet the headmaster. No further reference is made to Mrs Pearce's worries about how she can cope with Steven. The mediators feel that it is not part of their brief to act as social workers, although they are concerned about the difficulties facing Mrs Pearce. We leave.

Mrs Pearce does not make contact.

Totton Juvenile Court

The waiting room is packed full of children and parents, overflowing on to the landing. All have been called for 10 a.m. Only three cases are taken in the first two hours. It appears that they take the not guilty pleas first, presumably because these are the cases involving solicitors.

Mrs Pearce is losing money from her job as a van driver every minute that she's here. Because Stephen's case is not called until the end of the morning she will lose a day's pay.

12.45 p.m. Steven's case is the last to be called. He is un-represented. The clerk begins by asking Mrs Pearce whether she has received notice of her right to advance disclosure of the prosecution case. She says she hasn't. Does she want to exercise her right? No. Does Steven admit the charge? Yes. Does she accept that? Yes.

The prosecuting solicitor outlines the case against Steven. Two girls overheard his friend 'dare' him to smash the window. Then they heard the sound of breaking glass. Steven admitted to the police he'd done it. There is a compensation claim of £40.

Steven is asked if he'd like to say anything. He mutters a few words. He gives the impression that he could say something, if encouraged, but he's not encouraged. He's finding it very hard not to smile: a tense, nervous grin keeps breaking through. The whole performance – he and his mum, kitted out in their best gear, being addressed by this middle class woman – it's a bit of theatre in which he, a very inexperienced actor, appears to have been allocated a central role.

Mrs Pearce is asked whether she wants to say anything. She gives a delightfully naive performance. Steven has been getting into lots of trouble of late, she says. He must have broken the window deliber-ately, because that's the kind of thing he does. She doesn't actually say, as she'd said to the mediators, that she finds Steven a terrible problem and needs help in dealing with him, but that is the message behind her words. There is no probation officer in court; nor any representative of the reparation scheme. No mention is made of the abortive 'mediation'.

It is revealed that Steven has committed one previous offence – a minor theft 'a long time ago' for which he was cautioned. He is fined

£10 and ordered to pay £40 compensation. Mrs Pearce is asked how Steven proposes to pay. She says he's going to work part-time for his father, earning £5 per week. The chairman of the bench tells her that she will have to get this money from Steven. Meanwhile, responsibility for paying the fine and compensation lies with her. How soon can she pay – within fourteen days? She agrees to pay within fourteen days.

Case Two

Mr Rossi

Mr Rossi has been charged with stealing and falsifying a housing benefit cheque to the value of £127. This had been sent to a lodger of his, after he had left his premises. A meeting has been arranged between Mr Rossi and the Treasurer of the Local Authority Housing Department, a Mr Lovett. The meeting takes place in the offices of the housing department. The mediators are Carol (probation officer) and Barbara (volunteer).

The choice of 'victim' in this case is worthy of note. The Treasurer, of course, has suffered no personal loss. In so far as anyone did suffer personal loss, at least for a time, it was the rightful recipient of the benefit cheque. Mr Rossi's explanation for the theft, offered to the mediators beforehand, suggests, in fact, that a meeting with *the lodger* would have offered greater opportunity to explore the rights and wrongs of this case.

Before we are ushered in to see the Treasurer Mr Rossi nervously rehearses the arguments and justifications that he wishes to employ. He owns a cafe, with a bed and breakfast establishment upstairs. This is let to Supplementary Benefit claimants. Mr Rossi has now given up the bed and breakfast side, he tells us, because too many people left without receiving their benefit cheques and without paying any rent. Mr Rossi claims that the couple whose cheque he stole actually owed him more money than the amount of the cheque. He'd lent them £50 and had also allowed them to postpone rent payments. They had left owing large amounts of rent, having claimed that they were not getting their Benefit.

When we are ushered in to see Mr Lovett, Mr Rossi immediately begins to pour out his explanations, at the same time appearing extremely contrite. Mr Lovett intervenes at one point in order to establish that the envelope containing the cheque was clearly marked

– so Mr Rossi knew what he was doing, that is, tampering with someone else's mail.

Then we have a diversion as Mr Rossi and the Treasurer discuss another cheque sent to Mr Rossi's property – made out to the wrong person apparently – which Mr Rossi returned. This is Mr Rossi demonstrating that he's on the side of officialdom – distancing himself from the 'offender' role. He makes many and varied attempts to do this: (1) apology; (2) denial that this is his normal behaviour; (3) plea that he had been 'wronged' by the victim; (4) fact that he had taken another wrongly made out cheque to the police (so he's really a solid citizen); (5) describing how hard he works and how generous he's been to past lodgers (solid citizen again).

Barbara: He's been very worried actually, haven't you Mr Rossi?

Mr Rossi: I knew I done wrong. It was out of spite – I done it on the spur of the moment.

Barbara: The repercussions for Mr Rossi are quite serious. He lives in the community . . .

Mr Rossi: Yes, I know I done wrong, but I thought, quite honestly I was getting it out of (lodger). That's who I thought was . . . because he hasn't been anywhere near me since (to pay what he owes). My wife gave him clothes; we gave him free meals; there was a time he lost all his wages down the club playing cards, and if his wife had found out there'd have been a lot of trouble. We lent him £50 then to tide him over . . . you know, you just can't run a business like that. This is why we've packed it in – and just doing the cafe.

Mr Lovett explains that the council will only enforce payment to the landlord if a debt exceeds £500: 'not much consolation, I know.'

Mr Rossi: Several times I've written letters to Social Security, asking, when we had the flats, if they'd send the money to me. And they've said, no, that the cheque has to go to the person himself . . . I have to get up early in the morning . . . you know, it doesn't seem sort of right how they can't do nothing about it, with so much of it bleedin' going on.

(Sympathetic mutterings from Treasurer.)

Mr Rossi then offers to repay what he owes, by which I take it he means he could make out a cheque there and then. (Barbara had

discussed this point with the Treasurer beforehand. He had told her that
he did not feel able to accept payment before the court appearance.)

Barbara: I've explained to Mr Rossi that you're not in a position
to accept a cheque today, before the court meets, because, where it's a body rather than a private individual,
and it's a court case, you can't really set a precedent . . .
(Turning to Mr Rossi) It's new ground, so all that we
can do – and hopefully the court should be informed that
you've made the offer – and the Treasurer will say to
you that certainly he'd like the money as soon as possible, but after the court case . . .

Mr Rossi: Yes, certainly.

Barbara: In other words, that you can pay the full amount after
the court case, by a certain date.

Mr Lovett: Well, Mr Rossi, all I've . . . I've no further comments to
make about the matter . . . about the whole background,
as you'll appreciate.

Mr Rossi: Quite honestly, I knew I shouldn't have done it; I
shouldn't have opened it in the first place – no.

Mr Lovett: But I appreciate you coming to see me and I certainly
unreservedly accept your apology.

Mr Rossi: Thank you very much. It'll never happen again. It's not
my scene. I work from half eleven in the morning to
eleven at night. I was very surprised that they didn't . . .
when they first came to me, they looked pretty genuine
. . . they'd had a bit of a hard time you know, but I did
expect them really to come and pay, after all they owed
me, or some of it, but when they just . . . anyway . . .
(tails off)

Mr Lovett: OK? (as a signal for us to leave)

Barbara: Yes. Thank you. It's very kind of you, Mr Lovett, to
take this time, it is really.

Mr Rossi: Well, I do appreciate it.

Mr Lovett: I understand that. OK. Alright? (as a signal for us to
leave)

Barbara: Thank you. It's very kind of you indeed.

Mr Lovett: OK. Thanks very much indeed.

We all troop out (15 minutes approximately).

In the discussion afterwards Mr Rossi asks Carol (probation
officer) if she will speak for him in court. He feels he'll be

tongue-tied. He has not instructed a solicitor because he feels he can't afford the cost . . . although, he enquires anxiously, if it were a case of him getting six months . . . ? He is assured that the result ought to be a fine or conditional discharge. Carol says she will be present in court, but that the magistrates like the offender to speak for himself if possible. She will be ready to say something on his behalf, however, should he dry up.

Mediation report

A meeting took place on 19th January between Mr Rossi and Mr Lovett, Treasurer, — District Council in the presence of Mrs B.P —, Probation Volunteer and myself.

Mr Rossi had expressed a strong desire to apologise to the aggrieved party and also to repay the sum involved.

The meeting took place at the — District Council offices and was extremely cordial. Mr Rossi explained the circumstances of the offence and offered his apology to Mr Lovett. Mr Lovett said he accepted Mr Rossi's apology unreservedly and said he appreciated Mr Rossi's actions in coming to the mediation session.

Mr Rossi wishes to repay the amount involved in full, although it was agreed that in this instance it could be left to the court to make an order regarding compensation.

Totton Magistrates Court

10.30 a.m. Mr Rossi's case is called. He is unrepresented. He is charged with *two* offences: using a false instrument; and forgery. Clearly disconcerted by this, Mr Rossi (bravely) asks to speak, pointing out there was only one cheque. The two charges are, of course, a legal technicality. They either represent a pedantic approach on the part of the Inspector, or reflect police policy designed to boost clear-up rate.

Magistrate: Mr Rossi, have you sought legal advice? These are quite serious matters.

(No, he hasn't.)

The clerk to the justices then tries to persuade Mr Rossi that he should consult a solicitor. The probation officer (Carol) intervenes to say that a reparation report is available to the court.

Magistrate: It is essential that you have some legal advice.

The case is put back for Mr Rossi to consult the duty solicitor. He is clearly upset at this – he looks miserable and worried as he walks out of court.

The magistrates' insistence on legal advice could prove embarrassing for the reparation scheme should Mr Rossi change his plea to one of 'not guilty'.

10.55 a.m. The case re-starts, with the duty solicitor acting for Mr Rossi.

The prosecuting solicitor outlines the case. He mentions that the tenants had left still owing rent, but says that they had left furniture in lieu of payment. (This has not been mentioned by Mr Rossi.) He gives the police account of their interview with Mr Rossi – his explanations and justifications were dismissed as 'waffle'. The prosecutor does explain that Mr Rossi thought he was taking the money from his former tenant, rather than from the housing department – and that he did this because he thought he was owed money for meals and rent. He says that Mr Rossi has not repaid the housing department. He also refers to 'matters previously known' against Mr Rossi (unspecified).

The duty solicitor refers immediately to the reparation report – which the magistrates retire to read. When they return, the solicitor explains Mr Rossi's business. He says that he has suffered several instances of non-payment. The tenants from whom he stole the cheque had left without giving notice and without paying the rent they owed. At that point, 'temptation overcame Mr Rossi and he decided to re-coup his losses'. His one previous conviction was for theft of copper. The solicitor mentions Mr Rossi's apology to the Treasurer, and his willingness to repay the money, but doesn't say that he'd offered to do so before the hearing and that this offer had been declined. He asks for a Conditional Discharge.

It is noteworthy that Mr Rossi does not say a word throughout the proceedings. He is not asked to speak by the magistrates. (This doesn't square with the probation officer's previously expressed view that magistrates like the defendant to speak for himself.)

Mr Rossi is fined £50 on each charge – £100 in total. He is also ordered to pay the full compensation within 28 days. He asks for – and is granted – a further month.

Magistrate: Thank you for your help Mr — (duty solicitor). Thank you for your report (to probation officer).

No word is spoken to Mr Rossi, who looks bewildered for a few moments. Eventually he gathers that he's free to leave.

Afterwards, I ask Mr Rossi how he thought he'd been dealt with by the court.

Mr Rossi: Very fair, very fair indeed.

I: Did the visit to the Treasurer make any difference, do you think?

Mr Rossi: I think the report did, definitely. Because he accepted my apology and that must have gone in my favour.

I: What do you think of the reparation scheme?

Mr Rossi: I think it's a good thing, because I didn't know what to do, what to say – and the lady, she did stand up . . . she said I'd been to the meeting.

I: Any impression of the magistrates?

Mr Rossi: I wouldn't even recognise them. I know they don't come in our place and eat.

Case Three

Robin McDonald (15)
Robin is charged with theft of sweets to the value of 48p, taken from a large store in Totton.

Mr and Mrs McDonald are separated. Robin lives with his mother and three sisters. Mrs McDonald is sent the standard introductory letter.

Dear Mrs . . . ,
I understand your son Robin is due to appear in Totton Court on Wednesday 6th February. I should like to call and see you and Robin for an informal chat about this.

Perhaps I could call this Thursday, 22nd January at about 4.15 p.m. I will have a colleague with me.

I hope this is convenient and look forward to seeing you.
Yours sincerely,

Probation Officer

The visit to the offender

The case has been allocated to Norman (volunteer) and Carol (probation officer).

The three of us are welcomed by Mrs McDonald. She ushers her three daughters (all younger than Robin) out of the living room where they've been watching TV. Robin enters. He has a pleasant, open face. He says nothing. The mediators begin. Is he pleading guilty? Yes. Has he got a solicitor? No. They ask for an account of the offence. Robin gives it. He took two bars of chocolate. Then the mediators broach the subject of reparation – perhaps an apology to the store manager? How would Robin feel about that?

He replies: It's only 48p's worth.

This does not appear to be the right answer. Carol, who is doing all the talking at this stage, responds to the effect that, nevertheless, going to court is a serious matter and even if it was only 48p, it's still stealing. How would he feel about apologising?

Robin: I don't know, really.

Norman intervenes at this point: 'What's your feeling about the whole thing?'

No immediate response from Robin.

Norman tries again: 'Do you regret it?'

Robin: Oh, yeah (said with a reasonable degree of conviction).

Mrs McDonald intervenes. She starts to tell us, at some length, about Robin's dietary problem. He has been diagnosed as allergic to cocoa and dairy products. When he eats chocolate, he becomes 'hyper-active' – bad tempered, argumentative, difficult for her to control. But he also has a craving for the chocolate which has this effect on him.

Robin is then asked if he's been in trouble before. Yes, Mrs McDonald says, he began getting into trouble a few years ago. There's only been one *offence*, for which he was cautioned, but he's been getting into scrapes with other boys – trespassing and so on, thereby becoming known to the police. Again, she links this to the dietary problem – 'he couldn't settle; couldn't keep still.'

No word from Robin on diet; he doesn't confirm or deny his mother's account, and he's not asked. I suspect that at one stage he stops listening altogether – he seems in a world of his own.

Mrs McDonald embellishes her account. At one point, after consulting an allergy specialist, Robin gave up chocolate, cow's milk, etc. But then he started a paper round. He felt he should be able to do what he liked with his own money, so he went back to eating chocolate. His erratic behaviour resumed – 'he's got to be on the go'. Mrs McDonald is quite forceful – she complains at one point about the lack of facilities for youngsters in Totton. She comes across as a strong, determined woman.

The focus switches back to Robin. Carol asks about his previous offence. She emphasises the significance from the court's point of view of his previous caution. (This is her way of suggesting that he'd do well to take his position seriously – theft is serious, however small the amount.) She puts the proposal to him again, but without really clarifying the reasons why he should apologise. She doesn't say it would be a good thing in itself, but nor does she refer to the possible impact upon the court.

Robin responds: 'That's alright' (without enthusiasm).

Norman intervenes: 'How are you getting on at school?'

Robin responds: 'OK.'

Carol perseveres: 'Any favourite subjects?'

'Craft subjects,' Robin responds.

Norman: If you saw the manager of (store), what would you say?
What sort of promise would you make him?

Robin: I don't know, really.

Robin shows no sign of remorse at having taken the chocolate, although he's worried about what will happen to him. But in response to this minimal acquiescence it is taken that he has agreed to apologise, so the arrangements for this can go ahead. This is despite the mediators having failed to achieve any clear demonstration of appropriate attitude on Robin's part, which is what they were seeking at the outset.

Carol asks whether Mrs McDonald will accompany Robin when he meets the manager. Mrs McDonald says she wouldn't want to force herself on him. He's a very independent person. She also volunteers that he's had a lot of independence forced upon him (this statement is not elaborated). Robin says that he'd prefer to go on his own. He is asked if he's nervous at the idea of meeting the manager: 'A little bit.'

At the end of the interview Carol remarks that 'at least seeing the manager can't do Robin any harm' – the most direct reference to there actually being some inducement for him to make this apology. It has, I think, been implicit throughout, but the mediators have been striving to uncover other motivations.

Carol says she'll phone when she's spoken to the store manager.

We are unable to observe the meeting between the mediators and the store manager at which he agrees, after considerable initial reluctance, to meet Robin. Neither he nor his staff have done anything like this before.

The joint meeting

This meeting takes place in the store manager's office.

Present are: Carol and Norman (mediators); Robin; Mr Prior (manager); and researcher.

Carol makes the introductions. She explains that Robin has to go to court next week. She says that he 'would like to offer an apology and an explanation'.

All look at Robin.

Robin: I'm very sorry for taking the chocolate. It won't happen again. (Two short, well-prepared sentences.)

Mr Prior asks *why* he took them. Robin hesitates, then: 'My mates had some food and I didn't, and I had no money.'

This explanation appears to be accepted and Mr Prior launches into an account of the economics of a company such as this one and tries to explain the costs of shoplifting from the company's point of view. His explanation of company accounting is too complicated for me to follow. I don't know how Robin's managing – he looks completely out of his depth. The store operates on a stock-counting basis – so all goods must be accounted for; not on a *profit* basis, under which the manager is given a margin within which to operate.

Mr Prior stops suddenly in mid-explanation, just as he's saying: 'I can best explain this . . . if you're interested, are you?' Robin has obviously stopped listening and the manager's noticed it.

Robin mumbles assent.

Mr Prior tries again – and does a little better this time. He equates shoplifting losses to the wages of his staff: they lose the equivalent of four staff per annum. He implies that shoplifting is *costing jobs*. Robin's attention is caught.

Norman intervenes here (at some cost to the message which the manager is trying to convey) to suggest that many of the losses will result from *staff* theft. Mr Prior agrees. He now switches tack to talk of the costs to Robin of his going to court – this is 'very detrimental'. He says it is bound to affect the way in which he, an employer, would consider him as a job applicant. 'Then', Mr Prior goes on, 'if you get away with it for a while and it escalates, it could ruin your life.' Perhaps thinking that this sounds a bit dramatic, he adds: 'I'm not trying to put fear into you.'

Mr Prior's approach is stern but basically well-disposed: he's giving Robin a good talking to. He concentrates on the boy's own interests, rather than on moral principle.

Robin does seem to be listening. He's no longer off in a dream world. He acknowledges that the offence has damaged him. As Mr Prior puts it: 'It's another hassle you've got to overcome.'

Mr Prior then mentions the worry which the arrest and court appearance will bring to Robin's parents – 'you're letting them down as well'.

Norman at this point asks whether the manager 'has any attitude on Robin having come to see him?'

Mr Prior hesitates. He doesn't appear to be in an encouraging mood, although he recognises what is required of him. 'Well, yes, that's obviously commendable because, I suppose, you're making yourself target for tonight. Though it would have been even better if your parents had come here . . . ' The mediators appear nonplussed at this. Eventually Carol explains Mrs McDonald's reason for not coming, that is, Robin's desire to be independent. Robin also chips in to say that his mum has his three young sisters to look after. Mr Prior, still a bit grudging: 'Well, it's commendable and courageous to put yourself on the spot.'

Norman: So he gets a *little* plus. (He evidently thinks that Robin needs something more positive; he doesn't want him to feel he's just had a dressing down. Then, turning to Robin) 'Do you appreciate the attitude?' (Not clear if this means: do you get the point? – or, do you appreciate the manager's attitude towards you?)

Robin: Yes.

Norman: Would you like to tell him?

Robin: I appreciate your attitude.

Thanks all round. We leave. The mediators are pleased. They feel it's been a good meeting. They are especially relieved given the difficulty which they experienced in getting Mr Prior to co-operate.

There is now the prospect of securing further 'mediations' at this store.

Totton Juvenile Court

Robin's case is called at 12.00 noon – this is after he, his mother and father and four-year-old sister have been waiting for two hours.

The clerk asks Mrs McDonald whether she's had notice of her right to advance disclosure of the prosecution case. Consternation from Mrs McDonald – she's forgotten to bring the notice. Does she wish to exercise her right? No.

The prosecuting solicitor outlines the case against Robin. He's had *three* previous cautions, the last of which was in July 1984 (two and a half years ago). Presumably it is the three previous offences – however minor – which have brought him here on this charge of stealing 48p's worth of chocolate.

Robin is asked what he wants to say. He says he's sorry. The chairman of the bench intervenes: was he *hungry*? No, he'd eaten his lunch sandwiches.

Mr McDonald stands up at this point – unbidden – and asks if he can speak. He tells of the divorce – and of the bitterness between him and his wife over maintenance. This must have affected Robin, who is a good child at heart. (This is quite a moving speech in its way. He's taking the blame, in effect, and trying to shield his son.)

Then Mrs McDonald is asked if she wants to say anything. She explains Robin's diet problem. She has a sheaf of letters from the specialist. The magistrates ask whether Robin receives pocket money. She says he used to have a job, but not now. She doesn't mention the baby-sitting (which earns Robin money), but says he's a very helpful boy around the house.

The probation officer presents the reparation report – which, incidentally, has not been shown to Robin or his parents beforehand. A copy is passed to the McDonalds.

Robin is conditionally discharged for twelve months.

After court, I discuss the case with Robin and his mother.

I: What did you think of the way you were dealt with this morning?

Robin: I dunno . . . it was new . . . I presume those three people were sort of a jury . . .

I: Well, magistrates, but similar to a jury.

Robin: And I had to stand up every time I was questioned.

I: Very formal, did you think?

Robin: Yes, I didn't see much point in that really, but I suppose it didn't do me no harm.

I: Did you think they were sympathetic?

Robin: Yes, I think I was very lucky actually – I could have got something worse than that.

I: What about the (store) manager?

Robin: Well, very nice indeed actually. I thought he was going to have a go at me and . . . um . . . he educated me in what he said about jobs being lost and about my future . . . and things like that. I didn't know that what I'd done could lead to a big thing in his shop.

I: Could you understand what he was saying?

Robin: Yeah, he explained himself well.

I: Did you feel under pressure to go there?

Robin: Well, I thought it might, like, make a difference . . .

I: With the court?

Robin: Yeah, if I went to see him. I didn't think I was getting much benefit out of it, but it was an experience to go to see him . . .

I: Not a complete waste of time?

Robin: No.

I: Is shoplifting common amongst your friends?

Robin: No . . . well, it used to be. When we was young, we didn't have much money, we used to go in town purposely, for a nicking spree. We used to go in, get a load of stuff, come back home, say 'look what I got' and this sort of stuff. We got caught twice for that, in a big gang, then that was it, there was no more of it.

Case Four

Michael Morley (18)

This was the most serious offence in which the reparation scheme became involved during the period of our study. It may, indeed, have been the most serious over the life of the scheme since it was the only case in which the offenders were committed to Crown Court for sentence.

Michael and his co-defendant, Kevin Brown (who was remanded in custody) attempted, in two separate incidents, to snatch the handbags of two women. They were camouflaged, with balaclavas and other Army gear. They took one woman's bag. One of the victims, a Mrs Hall, succeeded in hanging on to hers, but fell to the ground in the scuffle.

The case is allocated to Carol (probation officer) and Annette (volunteer). They see no prospect of initiating mediation in the case of Kevin Brown (who already has a formidable criminal record) since he has been remanded in custody, but it is decided to attempt to engineer a meeting between Morley and the two women. We are unable to observe the preliminary visits to the victims because it is felt that, given the nature of the offences, it would be potentially upsetting to have three people (and one of them, a man) arrive on the door-step. In fact Carol and Annette decide not even to write a preliminary letter in this case. They are apparently well-received by both of the victims, but one – who is younger, and more upset by the offence – declines to meet Morley. The other victim, Mrs Hall, who succeeded in hanging on to her bag, agrees to meet him.

The meeting takes place in Hythe Probation Office. Mrs Hall arrives at the same time as me: we're ushered into a room where Carol, Annette and Michael are already seated. Michael is tall and well built (over 6 foot), tidily dressed, and looks chronically anxious and embarrassed. He can hardly bear to look up as the introductions are made.

Carol: Well it's really up to you, Mrs Hall, to have a word with Michael now.

(This is interesting. Why should it be up to Mrs Hall to begin?)

Mrs Hall starts, without any word having come from Michael. She is extremely voluble, appearing well in control of the situation. Her tone is reproachful, and yet sympathetic: 'I know how you feel – you must feel *terrible* (Michael mumbles assent) – but what on earth made you do it?! How would you feel if my son had done that to your mother?'

It emerges that Mrs Hall is separated from her husband and has a son Michael's age. Michael and Mrs Hall live on the same street and know one another by sight – or at least, she knows him.

Mrs Hall continues. She says that when she told other people who it was that had tried to snatch her bag, the response was one of shock – 'Oh no, not Michael.' She asks Michael (rhetorically) if he's ever

thought how this sort of thing makes a woman feel – 'It's only
because I'm a woman; it wouldn't have happened to a man.' She
stresses (several times) that 'it's a violation'. (Does Michael understand the point she's making? He gives no sign, although listening
closely. He is looking less embarrassed than at point of initial introduction, although clearly still in the dog-house.) Mrs Hall is doing all
the talking – no need for prompting from Annette or Carol. She is
remonstrating with Michael, but there is an undercurrent of kindli-
ness in her attitude towards him.

Mrs Hall: The first week (after it happened) I could really have
strangled you, but I'm over my anger – it's gone now – I
realise this is a one-off – that it won't happen again.

(Michael assents, although he hasn't actually said this himself. But his
whole attitude indicates contrition, and he has mumbled some
shame-faced words of apology as well as indicating assent at various
points in Mrs Hall's lecture.)
Mrs Hall repeats: 'I've lost my anger.' She asks again: 'What made
you do it?'

Michael: I was looking for a job, and I had no money. (He never
actually explains why, as a response to these difficulties, he
resorted to handbag snatching.) We didn't single you out
– it wasn't as if we were watching you. (This does not
come across as wholly spontaneous; perhaps it's a point
which the mediators had suggested Michael should make.)
Mrs Hall: It does make you feel better, knowing it wasn't personal.
Michael reinforces the point: 'We hardly seen you.'
Mrs Hall (who has now finished telling him off): I've got to be
honest, at no time did I feel *violently* threatened by you; there was no
time when I thought you were going to *be* violent.

(This is interesting: Michael is a big lad, and he and his mate were
camouflaged, but I can believe from her approach to this meeting
that Mrs Hall is not of a nervous disposition. The same may not be
true of the other victim.)
Michael confirms: 'That never even went through me mind.'
Mrs Hall refers back to the incident, almost with a touch of pride:
'But I wasn't going to let go.'

Annette intervenes at this point in order to switch the focus back to Michael: 'Would you like to tell Mrs Hall how you felt?'

Michael: I'm very sorry . . . and if there's anything I can do for *you*, like gardening . . .

Mrs Hall: Bless you (laughs).

Michael: My mum was devastated. It's the first time I've been in trouble with the police (not quite true, it emerges in conversation with me later: he'd been cautioned three years ago for shoplifting). I don't know what came over me.

Mrs Hall: I don't bear you any malice. I was very angry – I felt I really wanted to hurt you – not because I was physically hurt, but it was the *violation*. It's because you're a woman that it can happen to you . . . it's a sexual thing in that it's only something that a man would do to a woman.

Carol intervenes to remind Mrs Hall that she had been nervous for a while – 'looking over your shoulder'.

Mrs Hall: I'm not so nervous now, because I'm a reasonably strong character, but the old people (there is an old people's home in the same street), they're so nervous that they have to be escorted to the shops.

(This is a *major* consequence of the offence, if true, but no-one takes the point any further.)

Mrs Hall: I should imagine you feel a right idiot. I should hope you feel hurt for your mother's sake and for your own sake. I was imagining, if it was my son, I'd think 'how *dare* you!'

Michael has become visibly more relaxed through all this – the tone is not condemning of him as a person. He's still listening, however.

Mrs Hall: You put so much trust in your children, but when they do something wrong, you stand by them. I don't feel angry towards you now – my anger's gone. I wish you well . . . if there's anything I can do . . . (an interesting switch)

Carol: We'll be preparing a report for the court (implication: Mrs Hall already has helped Michael by agreeing to this meeting).

Mrs Hall: I hope you get yourself a job.

Michael then explains his efforts to get a job – first in Totton, then Hythe. This is the start of a fairly lengthy discussion of Michael's job prospects, signifying that: (a) the focus of the meeting is now on how to help Michael; and (b) the main problem he faces (and, by implication, the reason for his offending) is his lack of a job/money.

Mrs Hall: What about when you left school – did you have any help then?

Michael then takes us through his employment history: YTS; labouring jobs; made redundant; then unemployed for a few months; then labouring job on an industrial estate; sacked because of his time off, having hurt tendons in his wrist. He's been unemployed since October (five months). Has recently been for interview with a large store, but 'I was told I wasn't the right person at the right time, sort of thing. They're keeping my details, so they'll let me know if anything turns up.'

Mrs Hall: You could try TOPS – they'd give you training.
Annette: Is there anything you're interested in?
Michael: I'd thought of bricklaying . . .
Carol: It's quite hard to get on a bricklaying course.

(Interesting, the way this has gone: all three women are now working hard, trying to pool ideas as to how to help Michael find a job.)
    Michael himself contributes to the discussion (quite relaxed, accepting of their efforts to help him). He mentions a computer course which his mother had done. This would have cost him £20. Mrs Hall agrees as to the cost of all these courses. She'd thought of doing a cake icing course – but it would have cost her £65.

Annette: Perhaps you could have taken the plastering course and applied it to the icing.

(A modestly good joke, but I don't believe Michael got it. He refers, seriously, to watching plasterers at work when he had a labouring job. He saw someone getting in a stew because he couldn't manage it – which made him realise how difficult it was.)
    Mrs Hall talks of the need to get rid of excess energy: 'This is the trouble with boys, you know: they've nothing to do and then they get into trouble'.

Carol: If you've got all that excess energy, you could do some work for Mrs Hall. Would you like to do that?
Michael: I don't know as I'd like it, but I don't mind digging, mowing the lawn . . .

Mrs Hall: When the spring comes you can mow my lawn, *willingly.* (This is not said in the way of someone really expecting it to happen.)

Michael then tells us a bit about his lawn-mowing exploits: he is not a very distinguished exponent, apparently. Mrs Hall refers to the problems she's having with her garden. Annette chips in: amazing how long the grass kept growing this autumn; it was so mild leading up to Christmas. (Several minutes on this, Michael saying nothing, but no obvious signs of boredom or impatience. He appears mildly amused from time to time at things that are said. Mrs Hall and Annette are doing nearly all the talking, with Carol chipping in occasionally. All this is expressing relief that the meeting has gone well. There's an air of mutual satisfaction.)

Mrs Hall: (returning to Michael's offer of help) He only lives up the road, so if I want something I can shout 'Michael! Come and do this!'

Carol eventually brings this easy-going conversation to a halt: 'Well, you've had a long day at work (to Mrs Hall). Can I run you home?' Annette and Carol together: 'Thank you very much.'

Mrs Hall: I appreciate it very much. Earlier, I'd have had a real go at him. What's done is done. *You* realise (to Michael) what a big let-down it's been, more to *yourself* really.
Michael: And to a few other people. (Quite accepting this judgement, which is obviously critical, but proffered benevolently.)

Carol and Mrs Hall leave. I chat to Michael for a few minutes on my own. He expresses relief at the way he's been treated – 'I thought she'd have a go at me.' It seems that this expectation of being confronted by a vengeful victim, followed by a meeting with a real person who is *not* like that, can have quite a powerful effect, at least in the short term. It really does feel as if Michael has been forgiven.

Interview with Mrs Hall

I: How did you feel that evening – were you very upset?
Mrs Hall: Yes . . . to say I was upset (thinks) – I'm not a person that shows a great deal, but I just didn't go out . . . I can't say it upset me to the extent that I was sobbing or anything

like that. I just didn't go outside the door. The only time I went out was when I had to go to work. I didn't want to go out at all after that and luckily I had quite a few friends who picked me up – took me out and brought me home. It's only the last week or two that I've been going out unaccompanied again.

Mrs Hall then compares Michael's plight with that of her son – who persevered, under some difficulties, and in the end secured a decent job . . . 'I don't expect him to knock somebody about just to get some money, so that anger was still there, but equally, I feel sorry for him.'

Asked about the mediators:

Mrs Hall: They explained the situation. They said that Michael – it was a first offence – and they said: 'what did I feel about him?' . . . I'm glad I had the opportunity to talk to him because he (Michael) passed my gate about a week later and I wanted to go out and confront him and say 'this is me, and look at *you* – you're huge compared to me' – but that wore off, that was pure anger . . . And they (mediators) said, you know, how would I feel about meeting him, to accept his apology, and I said, yes, I *would* like to meet him.

I: For your own reasons, or did you feel it was something for him?

Mrs Hall: I think a bit of both – I wouldn't like to think . . . I think a first offence, everyone's entitled to a mistake in their life – unfortunately, he chose a really . . . not a very good one, but he doesn't seem a very strong boy mentally, and probably because my son is *so* strong-willed, he would never *ever* be led . . . I suppose I feel strongly for a kid who hasn't got that initial . . . (strength of character), so I can see that a child *could* be led by someone they think is a bit of a hard man – boys, they do go through these stages, and he's not a very mature boy, is he? But anyway, they just said – 'how would I feel?' – they didn't put any pressure on me; in fact, they kept stressing that I didn't have to; they didn't *want* to put any pressure on me . . . I don't *have* to go . . . and they told me that the other girl wasn't going – that she couldn't face him, so they were very open about it. I didn't feel obliged to go – if I wanted to go, then they'd be pleased, and if I *didn't* want to go, then there'd be no . . .

I: What did you think of Michael at the meeting?

Mrs Hall: (pause) Yes, I'll give him the fact that he had to face me, and I think that took courage, but I think maybe he was advised to . . .

I: Why?

Mrs Hall: Maybe to help his chances when it goes to court – I mean, I'm not unaware of that, and obviously this is what the probation office is all about, is to try and help these youngsters to have a start . . . I didn't think he was criminal material because I think he's too soft – and I don't mean that detrimentally to him. I just think his temperament is too soft. I think he's probably not very bright; I also think his mother hasn't probably helped him, because it seems to me – strength of character is starting something and finishing it – my son, I made it clear he had no choice (explains at some length her attitude to her son's working; his obligation to pay rent etc).

I: Did *you* get anything out of meeting him again?

Mrs Hall: I think I lost a lot of fear. I think I was probably frightened of coming face to face with him – perhaps not frightened, but worried, not knowing how to react if I did, because living up the road I'm bound to come face to face with him at some stage, and I wouldn't want to go up and say 'you're the one', you know (laughs). By that time, a lot of what I'd been feeling had gone . . . I'm not a weak character, but I know of a dozen others that would have been devastated by it. I think he was lucky he picked on me against somebody who wasn't the same temperament as myself.

I: He mentioned he'd do some gardening. Did you take that seriously?

Mrs Hall: If it makes *him* feel better, then he's welcome to have a go in the garden . . . if it makes *him* feel better.

I: It's not something you'd want for yourself?

Mrs Hall: I'm not bothered. I suppose in a way if it's therapy for him, to make him realise that hard work can overcome other things, then fine.

I: You wouldn't be afraid of having him around?

Mrs Hall: No! (laughs) My dog would have him if he even thought of touching me. (This is a joke, I think.) I don't think, had Michael really thought of it . . . he wasn't thinking logically at all, and I think he was just led. I would feel very upset if it was treated . . .

I: If he were sent to prison, for example?

Mrs Hall: That would really upset me – I really don't think Michael is prison material; I think *because* he's so easily led, I think he'd be better doing Community Service, or one of these new schemes that they give offenders . . . because I've got all my theories anyway . . . I think people what's on the dole should be made to do a day's work.

The report

1. Michael was approached by Mrs —, Voluntary Associate, and Mrs —, Probation Officer, to discuss this offence, and in the course of the interview he expressed remorse and a desire to meet the ladies concerned to apologise.

2. Having been allowed time to consider this prospect, one of the ladies decided, quite understandably, that she felt unable to meet with Michael but Mrs Hall agreed to do so and a mediation meeting was arranged for Thursday, 7th March.

3. During the meeting Mrs Hall conveyed to Michael just how she had felt both during and after the attack. She explained that she had initially felt angry and had for some time afterwards been reluctant to go out of her house. She was curious to know what Michael's motivation had been, and he was able to explain something about his own circumstances.

4. Michael apologised unreservedly for his behaviour and Mrs Hall accepted this. Both Mrs Hall and Michael expressed appreciation to the other for agreeing to the meeting. For his part Michael felt he had gained some insight into the personal impact of his action on his victims.

5. The meeting ended on a friendly and informal note with Michael offering to undertake any domestic chores Mrs Hall might require in reparation for the offence, and this was left as a possibility for Mrs Hall to consider.

Southampton Crown Court

Mrs Morley is present in court with Michael, as is the leader of the

Air Cadet Corps (from which Michael is suspended). Michael and his mother both appear desperately nervous: this sort of thing imposes a terrific strain, never mind the sentence. Carol (probation officer) remarks to me that she hopes Michael's brought his toothbrush – she expects him to be sent down.

Michael's co-defendant, Brown, is brought up from the cells and the two stand in the dock together. Mrs Morley and the Air Cadet Officer are on the public benches.

The prosecuting counsel says that Morley and Brown were 'on the lookout for an easy source of funds . . .'; they had intended to attack a jeweller's, but the obstacles had proved too formidable. Then they had tried to grab Mrs Hall's bag. The second offence occurred after they had been keeping watch on a cash-point machine in order to find someone to rob. They saw a young woman with her baby. Brown had wrestled her to the ground, whilst Morley had snatched her bag. Little of value was taken. The account of this robbery is presented in a flat, unemotional way, but the impression conveyed is of a very nasty, frightening assault.

A police officer gives Brown's antecedents: a long list, including two terms of imprisonment. He was sentenced in February (a month ago), for burglary with 49 t.i.c.s, to Two Years Youth Custody.

Brown is dealt with first. His barrister makes what he can of his client's co-operation with the police. He is being given training in prison – so that he can emerge with qualifications which will help him secure a job. Brown is only 17. He is already serving two years. The essence of the plea in mitigation is: what's the point of adding more on top?

Then Michael's barrister begins to speak. He refers at the outset to the Social Enquiry Report. The judge interrupts – 'a very persuasive one'. The barrister, slightly taken aback, says that he is heartened that his lordship takes this view. He resumes – only for the judge to interrupt again: 'Do you wish to try and improve upon it?' The penny drops. The judge is already persuaded, but is choosing this opaque method of conveying as much. Barrister: 'Then perhaps I needn't trouble your Lordship further.' Sits down. (He's only said about two sentences.)

Brown is sentenced to two years' imprisonment, concurrent with his earlier sentence, but starting from today. (That is, he gets an additional six weeks.) He is taken down.

The judge refers to Morley's age – eighteen. 'I've concluded, having read the Social Enquiry Report, and because of your age, it is not necessary to send you away.' He also refers to 'the account of an encounter with one of your victims'.

Michael Morley is placed on probation for three years. He is also ordered to pay £100 towards the prosecution costs. Counsel asks that he be allowed to pay at the rate of £10 per week.

Mrs Morley is sobbing uncontrollably at the side of the court. Michael walks from the dock and out into the court foyer, where he comforts his mother.

DISCUSSION

It will be apparent from the case studies that the Totton scheme operates in a way which is contrary to some of the most cherished tenets of reparation as practised at some other centres – notably those where the main object is to achieve diversion. At Totton the mediators seem quite prepared to take on cases where the offender is certain, in any event, to receive a low-level, non-custodial penalty from the court (the cases of Steven Pearce and Robin McDonald). The scheme's 1986 report acknowledged that they might do this *occasionally*, but as far as I could see they had few qualms about promoting what juvenile liaison bureaux might have termed 'an escalation of response'.

I do not necessarily see this as reason to be critical of the Totton scheme since the 'escalation of response' rhetoric obscures more than it illuminates. The question is, what *kind* of response – and what impact will different 'responses' have upon those who are subjected to them? A meeting with a store manager, in order to be informed about the impact of shoplifting on the economics of his business, is not to be equated with a period of Youth Custody. Robin McDonald may well have derived some benefit from his encounter. I did not feel, observing this, that he was being reinforced in a criminal identity. It was certainly nothing like a courtroom; 'authority' in this case was neither distant nor hostile.

Our time with the Totton scheme also enabled us to learn more about the question of offender *inducement* to make reparation, the understanding being that his or her efforts would be reported to a court. It seemed to us that the element of potential self-interest was perceived and understood by offenders and victims in all the cases which we observed. But having said that, there was still room for the offender's actions to be motivated, at least in part, by *contrition* (Michael Morley); and there was still room for the encounter with the victim to be *educative*, in the sense of promoting attitude change (Morley and McDonald).

The second caveat to be entered in respect of offender inducement (or self-interest) is that the impact of reparation on the sentence of the court appeared, in Totton as in Coventry, to be wholly uncertain. Michael Morley may well have secured a more lenient sentence through agreeing to meet Mrs Hall; but did Mr Rossi or Robin McDonald benefit in the same way through meeting their victims? Probably not. For McDonald to have received anything other than a conditional discharge would have been unthinkable, whilst only the most draconian magistrates would have imprisoned Mr Rossi for such a minor fraud. By the same token, would Steven Pearce (Case One) have been punished less severely had he apologised to the headmaster? We cannot tell, but in terms of limiting the overall cost and inconvenience to himself it is quite possible that he made the right decision. So there is a paradox: the mediators (at Totton as at Coventry) are reluctant to acknowledge the possible impact of reparation on the court sentence; nevertheless, this mitigatory potential is never denied – and our impression is that it is an important selling point – whilst the reality appears to be that this selling point (which does not need to be sold *hard* in order to be effective) is barely justified by the wholly unpredictable impact of reparation on the sentence of the court. It is potentially mitigatory, no doubt, but because sentencing is so erratic in any event there is no way of knowing what impact, if any, an act of reparation will have in a given case.

At Totton as at many other centres it is only *one form* of reparation which is being fostered – that is, explanation and apology. Other forms of making amends, such as immediate financial compensation, or work for the victim, do not appear to be seriously considered. I am not suggesting that non-material reparation is of little value: it may be a very important component in reparation – perhaps the most important, as with the Michael Morley case, but it is certainly not the *only* component, as the practice of the Totton and Coventry schemes might lead one to suppose. The form of reparation which has been developed in Totton reflects the scheme's relationship to the court, the time-scale within which it has to operate, and, thirdly, the kind of transactions which the mediators are comfortable with or have an interest in promoting. This third element is reflected, for example, in the scheme's interest in offender education – particularly the education of juvenile offenders. This is only reparative in the rather tenuous sense that, if successful in promoting offender attitude change, victims may have reason to be reassured that their rights will be respected in future.

The scheme's relationship to the court is obviously a potent influence. It has the result, in Totton as elsewhere, of downplaying *victim* interest in reparation. The format employed in the reparation report is itself a clear indication of this. This report is modelled on the traditional Social Enquiry Report. It gives the address, age, school or occupation *of the offender* – nothing about the victim. This in turn is a reflection of the fact that the court's responsibility is to punish the offender, not to deliver justice between citizens. The question of *how serious was the loss* (say, to the store manager in the McDonald case, or to the Local Authority in the Rossi case) did not form part of the subject matter of the report.

The fact that, in the mediators' preliminary discussion with offenders, reparation was almost invariably presented in terms of *an apology* was a reflection of the clear allocation of blame implicit in the 'crime' label having already been attached to one party's behaviour. We noted one case in Totton where the offender blamed the victim, at least in part, for what had occurred; as a result he was not prepared to apologise. He was not invited, as far as we are aware, to engage in a discussion of his responsibility relative to that of the victim, although one might infer from his initial response that this would have been much more acceptable to him.

The Rossi case presented another illustration of this pattern. It would not be fair to blame the Totton mediators, since they operate within a framework determined by their relationship to the court, but this was an excellent illustration of, in mediation terms, missing the point. There was a real issue of justice in this case, according to Mr Rossi. Of course we only heard his side of the story – but then it would have been interesting to hear that of his former tenants. Such an encounter, one imagines, would have had some meaning. Whether this 'meaning' could have been recognised by a court, Mr Rossi having been charged with a criminal offence, is a separate and difficult question: our criminal courts operate in such a way as to exclude all civil justice considerations. But the meeting with the Borough Treasurer might fairly be characterised as *a performance*. From the point of view of the mediators this case served to re-establish the scheme in the eyes of the court after a gap of several months; for Mr Rossi, there was the hope that his apology to the Treasurer might lead to a reduced sentence; but the justice issues in the case remained unexplored. Admittedly Mr Rossi's arguments and justifications were heard – both in the meeting with the Treasurer and in court – but the other key protagonist was not present on either occasion. There was a plea of mitigation, but the whole court appearance was stereotyped and sterile. This may be considered particularly unfortunate given that this case was well capable of being re-drawn in terms of dispute.

The evidence which we gathered at Totton (as at other centres) did not suggest that the scheme had a significant impact upon the practice of the local court. This was partly a reflection of the limitations imposed by criminal law and court procedure, but it also reflected what one might characterise as a failure of imagination (or lack of will) on the part of professional practitioners. We came across several indications of this – from magistrates, clerks, police, and the mediators themselves. All claimed to support reparation – but in a form which could easily be accommodated within, and would not seriously disturb, the practice of courts. For example, one magistrate at Totton argued that he could not permit reparation to be pursued too enthusiastically because he had a duty to protect the citizen and to express public standards. This of course raises a number of interesting questions. For example, how does he know that he *is* protecting? Is he sure that the punishments which he inflicts reflect community sentiment? Does the level of pain delivered in a given case convey the right moral message? In what sense can reparation be said to undermine morality; fly in the face of public opinion; or expose citizens to greater risk? Nevertheless, this was the view of reparation implicit in many of the comments made to us. At its heart lay a self-fulfilling prophecy: reparation is primarily 'symbolic' and designed to mitigate; if pushed too far, this could threaten the principles of community protection and proper punishment; so reparation must not be pushed too far.

I have yet to refer to the one outstanding example of effective mediation (and probation) practice which we came across whilst observing the Totton scheme. The Michael Morley case, it seemed to us, was a successful intervention on several counts. It was especially interesting because the fact of Michael acting, in part, out of self-interest (to improve his chances in court) did not prevent, or even hinder, the achievement of several other goals pursued by the scheme. In order to develop this point about the different levels of achievement in this case it may be helpful to enumerate the principal objectives of mediation and reparation schemes as these have emerged in the course of our investigations. Different schemes have different priorities, but the following list encompasses all the main goals:

1. On behalf of the victim, to 'heal the hurt' by providing explanation and apology and by challenging stereotypes.
2. To provide compensation – either through work or money.
3. On behalf of the offender, to divert from prosecution or to mitigate the court's penalty.
4. To promote learning or attitude change (and thus to discourage future offending).
5. To enable the offender to express sorrow or regret, thus allowing the possibility of being forgiven.

Let us compare the Rossi, McDonald and Morley cases in respect of these criteria. It is possible to construct a table, as follows:

Objective	Rossi	McDonald	Morley
1	No	No	Yes
2	No	No	No
3	?	No	Yes
4	No	Yes	Yes
5	No	No	Yes

Concluding thoughts

Our brief glimpses of the Totton magistrates court demonstrated quite strikingly the way in which the offender, as well as the victim, is denied effective participation in the justice process. In terms of 'crime control as drama' (Christie 1986) these cases were not a success. The offender was denied anything other than token participation in the stylised series of communications which took place in the courtroom. Even the plea of mitigation, whilst it referred to the offender's background, did not challenge his outsider status. In fact, through its being delivered by a representative, it tended to confirm it.

The Totton mediators hardly deserve to be criticised for failing to challenge the assumptions underlying the delivery of justice in our criminal courts. But the fact that reparation schemes do not achieve this in their own practice is certainly worthy of note. Courts are not interested in assessing relative responsibility or in hearing alternative accounts of the offender's behaviour. Awkward questions, such as whether the conduct in question is really as bad as is being portrayed, are not on the agenda. But one might have imagined that reparation schemes *would* have these questions on the agenda. In practice, however, they find this difficult. To question the allocation of responsibility implied in the 'victim' and 'offender' labels, and in the offence designation, would be time-consuming and contentious. It would also threaten these schemes' relationship to the court. The only lifeline available is to do (and think) as the courts do and think. Reparation schemes have to demonstrate that what they are trying to do will not undermine what the courts are trying to do. One way of characterising the resulting accommodation (exemplified by cases such as that of Mr Rossi) is to see courts as concerned with efficient processing, or through-put; reparation schemes as promoting 'symbolic' acts of reparation, or performances; and *no-one* as concerned to examine the offender's behaviour in the light of valued principles of justice. Because these schemes wish to secure acceptance by the court they concentrate on offender education. Secondly, they encourage offender performances which, whilst they may be viewed with some scepticism, cannot be entirely dismissed since they suggest attitudes (of contrition and acceptance of responsibility) which are traditionally rewarded within the retributive framework. It is only very occasionally, as in the case of Michael Morley, that we get a glimpse of the central role which reparation *might* play in our justice system – and of how powerful that would be.

Chapter 6

Dominant themes
Diversion and mitigation

The principal raison d'être of the mediation schemes whose practice we observed was not reparation by offender to victim, but, on behalf of the offender, diversion from prosecution or mitigation of the court's penalty. This dominant motif was not always acknowledged with complete frankness by those responsible for managing these initiatives, but it emerged clearly enough from the practice. In some instances, indeed, it seemed to become more pronounced over the life of the scheme as staff lost faith in reparation as a 'good' in itself. Several reparation schemes had altered their focus with diversion or mitigation in mind.

The emphasis on diversion is understandable if we remember that these experiments took place against a background of rapid growth in pre-court decision-making in juvenile justice (Pratt 1986; Davis et al, 1989). As Pratt observes, dispensing juvenile justice has become, for the most part, an administrative rather than a judicial task. At some centres, indeed, the juvenile court has been rendered almost redundant (Giller 1986). This trend has been given formal encouragement by the Home Office in a series of discussion papers (see, for example, Home Office 1984). The policy of diversion has, in turn, contributed to a steep decline in the number of custodial sentences passed on juvenile offenders (from 6,800 in 1983 to 4,000 in 1987). One feature of this growth in administrative decision-making has been the development of a complex tariff of pre-court disposals. Thus, juvenile offenders who come to the attention of the police for a second, third, or fourth time may still not be required to attend court; however, they may well be required to submit to an 'enhanced' police caution under which they engage in some activity or render some service. This, then, is one circumstance in which reparation may be encouraged; it is not reparation to or for the victim, except perhaps incidentally; instead, reparation is pursued in the service of diversion (Davis et al, 1988).

This approach was exemplified in the practice of some Juvenile Liaison Bureaux. Initially they had been persuaded of the value of reparation in its own right, but they came to give more and more emphasis to its diversionary potential. The interesting thing about Juvenile Liaison Bureaux, in this context, is that their staff (or at least, the non-police members of their staff) hold strongly to the view that we both prosecute and lock up far too many young people. As far as they are concerned, diversion makes sense *irrespective* of any attempt at 'offence resolution'. And yet they still find it necessary in some instances to bolster the case for diversion on the basis that 'reparation' will be made. This suggests that somebody needs to be appeased, that 'somebody', presumably, being the police, magistrates or judiciary. So diversion needs to be sold according to the values espoused within our predominantly retributive criminal justice system. It needs to be demonstrated (or at least suggested) that the offender has *suffered* and/or that he is *reformed*. Hence reparation.

Although reparation figured quite prominently in the approach of the Exeter Youth Support Team, some Juvenile Liaison Bureaux had determined, after an initial flirtation with the concept, to abandon it altogether. For example, the Northampton Bureau, whose practice we studied over several weeks (Davis et al, 1989), made it clear to us that they regarded their written policy on reparation as being out of date. They argued, citing Blagg's research into the neighbouring Corby Bureau (Blagg 1985), that juvenile offenders are rarely in a position to be able to offer financial compensation; that the victims of juvenile offenders tend to be corporate, so that a meeting between victim and offender is likely to be less relevant in any event; and that given the power imbalance between a juvenile offender and an adult victim the exercise may be experienced by the offender as further punishment (something that the JLB would not wish to support). Thus, the staff of the Northampton Bureau no longer saw it as part of their responsibility to mediate between victim and juvenile offender, or to promote reparation to the victim. The reparation option still attracted the police constable members of the team, but not their probation or social work colleagues. In general, because their commitment to diversion was overriding, this JLB contacted victims only where staff believed the offender to be at such extreme risk of prosecution that an act of reparation was the only thing that might sway the balance. Retributive justice was kept at bay (quite successfully, it seemed to us) but nothing was put in its place.

While staff of some Juvenile Liaison Bureaux were prepared to dabble in reparation (Exeter was much more enthusiastic than most) the majority held to a utilitarian conception of criminal justice which discouraged this form of intervention (and, indeed, most others). They maintained, following the tenets of labelling theory as advanced by Becker (1963), Lemert (1967) and Schur (1973), that the criminal justice process only served to confirm the young person in his or her criminal identity and offending behaviour (see also Davis et al, 1989). At some centres (although not Exeter) staff commitment to this conception was exemplary. They also showed considerable courage in sticking to their guns when (as was inevitable) they encountered police resistance in individual cases. But of course they rejected an *alternative* radical conception, which is that of justice expressed in terms of making amends. Instead, they dealt in standardised formulae: categories of crime; categories of response. They were not interested in unravelling the 'meaning' of the behaviour in question – to the offender, the offender's family, friends, neighbours – or, indeed, to victims. They preferred to work within objective criminal justice categories. This was because they were concerned to slow progress up the tariff – and so they dealt in the language of the tariff in order to achieve this (indeed, they tended to add to that language). But they were not interested in ideas of fairness, or in responding in ways that made sense to the parties. In fact, they had no faith in responding in any form.

Christie suggests that preoccupation with utilitarian punishment leads to perpetual dissatisfaction with our criminal justice system (1982, pp. 103 ff). (What we have does not seem to work very well, so we need more.) 'Within penal law, this leads to an everlasting demand for more punishments carried out by representatives who – rightly in the impossible situation in which they are placed – perceive themselves as a buffer between a savage population filled with lust for vengeance and some misfits in need of protection against receiving too much pain . . . ' This could be taken as a description of the more ideologically pure Juvenile Liaison Bureaux. Christie's account is illuminating because it explains the genesis of the diversion strategy. It also reveals this to be conservative. The JLB approach reflects a professional insight – that they are operating within a treatment and deterrent system which does not work – so they seek to mitigate its effects and generally undermine its logical outcome, but *not* to develop new ways of thinking about justice and pain delivery. As a result they are driven to operate a closed system of justice which takes no account of the reactions of either parents or victims.

Pre-court reparation schemes, such as the one at Exeter, are also in large part driven by their adherence to the diversion principle, while court-based schemes, such as those at Coventry and Totton, had mitigation at or near the forefront of their thinking. There was an obvious wish to influence the court – and to influence it in one direction only. Where mediation was attempted prior to the defendant's initial court appearance, as at Totton, an offender's *refusal* to meet the victim was never reported to the court: only positive messages were allowed to get through. The Coventry scheme, which operated on adjournment, had to prepare a report in these circumstances, but this was invariably couched in carefully neutral terms which glossed over the offender's refusal to co-operate, failure to keep appointments, etc. If a meeting had taken place, this was invariably written up in such a way as to present the offender's motivation and behaviour in the best possible light. These reports sought to convey an impression of neutrality – see also Young's account (1987) of the practice of the Wolverhampton scheme – but material which might convey an unfavourable impression of the offender was excluded or glossed over, whilst considerable significance was attached to the most perfunctory act of reparation.

THE PROBLEM OF INDUCEMENT

The reparation literature in the UK has been notably confused on the matter of inducement. In the early days the prevailing view appeared to be that reparation (which was almost entirely *non-material*) had to be altruistic in order to be worthwhile. The National Association of Probation Officers observed that 'where coercion is either implied or actual, then the notion of reparation is stripped of meaning' (NAPO 1985). It must be apparent, however, that there is an immense problem in seeking to reconcile state prosecution of an offence with the offender's freedom to choose to make reparation. Mediation schemes, nearly all of which seek to influence prosecution or sentencing decisions, struggle with this problem, sometimes in quite ingenious ways, but they cannot resolve it. So long as the offender's altruistic participation is so highly regarded, it is virtually impossible to locate these schemes within a retributive system. When diversion from prosecution or a reduced court penalty is contingent upon the offender's making reparation, altruism and contrition are called into question; the possible ulterior motive is all too plain to see.

The problem lies in seeking to influence the prosecution decision, or the sentence of the court, whilst at the same time aspiring towards attitude change, reconciliation, and absence of coercion. The criminal justice system is concerned, above all, with imposing appropriate retribution. It may, at a pinch, be prepared to take apology and material reparation into account, but the offender's motivation for those acts can seldom be established unequivocally. A sincere desire to make amends and a *requirement* to do so are not incompatible in themselves, but it is difficult to demonstrate that sincerity when the element of compulsion, or inducement, is introduced. It is hardly surprising, in these circumstances, that some victims were dubious about an offender's motivation in seeking to meet them (Young 1987).

To point out these difficulties is not to be cynical about the possibility of altruistic reparation. That would of course be the strength of any mediation scheme which operated independently of the criminal justice system. But one cannot expect offenders to be disinterested given the strenuous efforts which *are* made to persuade prosecutors or courts to take account of whatever vestigial element of reparation has been performed. This has led some leaders of the reparation movement in the UK to argue that mediation should indeed be 'separated from the criminal justice process, so that the opportunity for reconciliation between victim and offender would be entirely unconstrained . . . the offender should not feel constrained into admitting guilt and taking part reluctantly in mediation by the prospect of risking a custodial sentence otherwise' (FIRM 1986). But FIRM is, perhaps unsurprisingly, not consistent in its approach to this question. One of the authors of the above document was Tony Marshall, who has observed elsewhere that 'even a contrite offender may need some form of "carrot" to engage in what can be a challenging and embarrassing process' (Marshall 1986).

Our research gave us some clues as to whether a possible sentencing discount need undermine the value of non-material reparation expressed through meeting, listening, and perhaps expressing regret. We do not think it does so necessarily, as the case of Michael Morley, presented in Chapter 5, confirms. That there was an element of self-interest in Morley's agreeing to meet Mrs Hall is undeniable (and he did not attempt to deny it); but it seemed to us that this encounter nevertheless had therapeutic worth – Michael and Mrs Hall were each accepted and understood by the other.

Nevertheless, inducement is perceived to be a problem – a problem for courts and victims (because they cannot judge whether expressions of remorse are genuine) and a problem for offenders (who struggle to convince). Schemes adopted various strategies to deal with the difficulty which they perceived in selling that somewhat dubious product: non-material reparation performed under the inducement of a sentencing discount. Exeter, for example, told us that 'if a child or parent refuses to participate, the caution is administered and that is the end of the matter'. But an element of ambiguity remained in that it was further observed that the offender 'will have had an indication at the caution stage that someone will visit to discuss reparation'. We observed one caution at Exeter during which the offender was given an unmistakable message that reparation was an integral part of the cautioning mechanism. We would not be surprised if juvenile offenders in these circumstances regarded reparation (albeit confined to an apology) as binding upon them, even in the absence of formal compulsion. Court-based schemes were faced with similar dilemmas, albeit at a later stage of the justice process. Most admitted concern lest the offender agree to take part 'for the wrong reason'. Some tried to deal with this by stressing to the offender that an act of reparation would not *guarantee* leniency on the part of the Court (as indeed it did not).

Another way in which schemes tried to get round the problem of inducement was to employ enthusiastic volunteer mediators who were not steeped in the probation service ethos of diversion or mitigation, but who believed in reparation as a means of promoting attitude change, reconciliation, and the alleviation of victim loss or suffering. This enthusiasm for reparation led some mediators to deny altogether the mitigatory potential of the offender's participation in their scheme. For example, a mediator at Leeds told us that if he thought an offender was under the impression that an agreement to make reparation would influence the court, he would 'squash that thought immediately'. Similarly, a Southampton-based mediator told us that he would impress on victim and offender that their discussion was 'private' (despite the fact that it would subsequently be reported to a court). Richard Young, when researching the Wolverhampton scheme, likewise observed that project staff presented their role as simply that of effecting reconciliation between offender and victim;

the court was depicted as having the entirely separate task of meting out punishment (Young 1987). This attempt to fudge the diversionary or mitigatory potential of a reparative act is implausible and cannot be sustained. One potential benefit of reparation is its contribution to a justified restoration of trust. Given the relationship between mediation schemes and the courts, this contribution is bound to be of variable quality. We can hardly deal with this by denying offenders access to the information that an act of reparation may reduce the level of retribution imposed. That is both impracticable and a very paternalistic approach to adopt towards people who are supposed to come to share our moral values.

At Exeter we observed one encounter between a member of the Youth Support Team and a young offender which struck us as particularly capricious and unfair. The social worker concerned was attempting to probe the youth's motives (he had indicated, with great reluctance, that he was prepared to apologise to a rival group of lads who had been assaulted) when it was all too apparent that he did not consider that he had behaved wrongly according to his own code, and that therefore the only conceivable reason for apologising was to avoid prosecution. Because this lad was not a very effective dissembler, he failed the test. As the social worker observed: 'It looks as if you want to apologise for the wrong reasons'. But it is paradoxical that offenders be rewarded for making reparation on the basis that they did so without hope of reward. It would appear in that case that a scheme has to hide its diversionary or mitigatory intent from the offender, and be able to convince police and courts that it has succeeded in doing this, in order to maximise its diversionary or mitigatory potential.

Staff at the Coventry scheme were well aware of the problem of inducement and, as a corollary, impure motives. As we saw in Chapter 4, they sought to overcome this through rigorous testing of the offender's motivation and attitudes. In doing so, they were themselves manipulative. It was apparent that offenders accepted referral to the scheme in the hope of a sentencing discount. (Indeed, they may well have feared *additional* penalty were they to decline.) They were then subjected to disquisitions on the theme of choice ('I'm very concerned that it should be your decision'), perhaps repeated over several visits. They were, by that stage, in no position to reject whatever form of reparation was proposed. It seemed to us that there was an element of dishonesty in these exchanges, dishonesty which could not be laid at the door of the offender.

MATERIAL OR NON-MATERIAL REPARATION?

As we have seen, the reparation which is encouraged by practitioners within reparation schemes in England and Wales is almost entirely non-material. In many instances, indeed, it is limited to a formal expression of regret. This may be delivered face to face, or by letter. It is hardly surprising in these circumstances that there is concern about inducement and insincerity. According to Howard Zehr, these same anxieties are not nearly so prevalent in the USA where crime is seen as creating an obligation upon the offender and reparation is geared to the victim interest, commonly taking the form of work or financial compensation (Zehr 1986). Young's research on victims and offenders attending Coventry and Wolverhampton reparation schemes indicates that both groups were sceptical about the value of apology linked to a sentencing discount (Young 1987a). In his report on the Wolverhampton scheme Young suggests that 'if the scheme is to continue with its present emphasis on communication rather than (material) reparation, it would enjoy a good deal more support from victims and offenders if the intervention were to occur after sentencing had taken place' (Young 1987, p. 72).

This is not to suggest that reparation should be seen as residing solely in the offer of restitution. When an offence is committed, the harm done is never confined to damage to property, or to people's bodies; it also involves damage to a social relationship (Watson et al, 1989). So reparation, if it is to be complete, must include some attempt to make amends for the victim's loss of the presumption of security. An apology, or expression of regret, may go some way towards achieving this. However, the practice which we observed had two major weaknesses. First, as already discussed, an apology delivered in the context of criminal proceedings is an ambiguous sign of attitude change. This need not reflect bad faith on the part of the offender; it is an inevitable product of the situation. As Blagg recounts, having observed several apologies delivered through the Corby Juvenile Liaison Bureau: 'The apology fulfilled their (the offenders') expectations; they were punished by an authority figure; they were powerless to prevent the process; they acquiesced; they then, in order to retain peer-group status and keep their egos intact, retrospectively recreated the encounter as one in which sullen obeisance was transformed into heroic resistance' (Blagg 1985). The encounters which we observed were not all as grim as this, but an element of performance was evident in most of them. The other difficulty, and a curious blind-spot manifested by virtually all UK reparation schemes, is that in a context in which restitution is practically feasible for the offender, but remains undone, it is difficult to see how an apology could be thought sincere or reconciliation achieved. As Adrian Thatcher has explained, verbal expressions of regret are unlikely to be credible (or 'satisfactory') unless accompanied by longer term, non-verbal, tangible expressions of regret. Remorse has to be expressed through the totality of behaviour (Thatcher 1991).

Where the offender is not remorseful, as where restitution is feasible but not forthcoming, such restitution may need to be imposed. In that case reparation *would be the punishment* (either in whole or in part); it would not be undertaken with a view to mitigating the 'real' punishment, the latter imposed in a different forum, by sentencers operating on different principles. Such a proposal takes us a long way from the practice of UK reparation schemes, but that is inevitable. The present focus upon apology is highly questionable, as is the premium placed upon 'voluntariness'. There is a lack of realism and genuineness about many of these encounters and this is colluded at by mediators who deliberately suspend disbelief.

THE THREAT OF 'DOUBLE PUNISHMENT'

The reluctance to arrange (or even to contemplate) material reparation can be understood by reference to two abiding preoccupations of reparation schemes in England and Wales. Although separate, they are each held to constitute a threat of 'double punishment'. In this chapter I have been concerned with schemes' diversionary or mitigatory intent, but there is also, of course, considerable interest in reparation as something worthwhile in its own right. However, it is feared that reparation may: (1) unreasonably increase the burdens placed upon an offender in response to a given transgression; and (2) constitute an escalation of response (in a world in which responses are finely graded) so that the offender moves up the punishment ladder more rapidly than he would otherwise do. Because of these fears, pre-prosecution schemes aim to provide reparation on a basis of minimum intervention, once the alternative responses of no further action, an informal warning, or a police caution have been exhausted. Thus they discourage reparation by first time offenders, or reparation undertaken in response to minor transgressions. The Corby Juvenile Liaison Bureau told us that part of the thinking behind their decision to operate on a pre-court basis was the wish to avoid reparation being used as a sentencing option in a way that would represent 'well-intentioned but counter-productive additional impositions for the offender, rather than clear alternatives'. This suggests that Juvenile Liaison Bureaux (in common with the reparation schemes which we observed) are not committed to the view that victims have a *right* to reparation, or that offenders are under a corresponding *obligation*. Nor do they feel bound to consult victims about the decisions being made in these cases.

The fear that offenders may suffer additionally has led pre-prosecution schemes to worry lest reparation be performed and the offender still be prosecuted, whilst court-based schemes are concerned lest reparation be undertaken and the offender be granted no reduction in sentence. This highlights the difficulty of seeking to operate systems of reparative and retributive justice side by side. It is especially problematic given the premium currently placed on absence of coercion within the reparative framework and on the imposition of appropriate levels of pain within the retributive framework. These difficulties remained unresolved in the practice of the reparation schemes which we monitored. For example, we observed several cases at Coventry and Totton where it seemed highly probable that reparation (invariably of a non-material kind) failed to achieve a sentencing discount. In these cases, even if the burden was minimal, it was extra. This arose in part because these schemes were seeking to build up their workload, and in part because they did not entirely accept the 'double punishment' argument; in other words, they had some commitment to a competing principle, this being that reparation was an appropriate obligation to place upon the offender. We were told at Totton that only very occasionally did the mediator suggest reparation in a case where the offender was likely, in any event, to receive a low level, non-custodial penalty from the court. It seemed to us, however, that the restrictive offence criteria under which this scheme was operating (low tariff, basically) meant that this was precisely the kind of case which they were likely to get.

The only evidence of 'double punishment' which involved material reparation (and no apparent sentencing discount) was supplied to us by the Leeds scheme. They described one case in which the offender had pleaded guilty to two charges: (1) burglary of school premises; and (2) arson of a car. An agreement was reached between offender and victim in both cases. In the first, there was an apology, coupled with an offer to repair broken goal posts at the school. This latter task was completed. The offender, who was a joiner, had also offered to make toys for the parent–teacher association. With respect to the second offence, the offender had apologised and agreed to pay compensation at the rate of £10 per week to cover the cost of a replacement car. In the event, he was given a 12 months' Youth Custody sentence. The Leeds co-ordinator commented that the victims saw this as inappropriate given the element of reparation that had already taken place, and certainly it was not what the mediator had wanted.

But I would not wish to convey the impression that, in general, reparation schemes contributed to an escalation of response, either resulting in additional burdens on the offender or accelerating his or her move up the tariff ladder. The emphasis on diversion was much too strong for that, particularly in the case of Juvenile Liaison Bureaux. It is more important to point out that 'double punishment' or 'escalation of response' is not in itself a very sophisticated notion. It surely matters what *kind* of response. Making amends could prove a positive experience for the offender; it is not necessarily to be equated with a court appearance, or being sent to prison. To this extent the whole notion of 'diversion' gives rise to some unease. Diversion from what, and to what? Our criminal courts may display an unduly restricted conception of justice, but presumably we would not wish offenders to escape justice altogether. Unfortunately, this is the impression created by those reparation schemes which have diversion or mitigation at the forefront of their thinking. If an act of reparation were viewed as part of the justice process, then it would make no sense to talk in terms of 'diversion'.

REPARATION IN THE SERVICE OF DIVERSION OR MITIGATION

On the basis of the picture presented so far, it can be seen that many reparation schemes are mis-described in that their principal objective is not reflected in their title. Diversion from prosecution or mitigation of the court's penalty cannot in themselves make good the harm done, so schemes having this as their *main* aim are better not described as reparation schemes; they are primarily concerned to achieve disposals least restrictive of the rights of offenders. Second, there is no necessary connection between reparation and diversion; pursuit of reparation *in the service of diversion* is a reflection of the huge shadow cast by our retributive criminal justice system. Any new initiative taken in respect of offenders is likely to be used (and abused) in this way. This is because all those involved – including sentencers themselves – are desperate to discover additional options which might permit them to mitigate the destructive effects of a retributive system.

The fact that these two concepts are linked in this way, with reparation essentially subordinate, can only serve to undermine the development of reparative justice. Reparation is being tacked on to our existing criminal justice system: it may increase the extent to which remorse and restitution are taken into account by sentencers, but we are not, as yet, moving towards a justice system in which private conceptions of the harm done and of what might be done to make it right weigh very significantly alongside the state-imposed tariff. Paradoxically, the diversionary objective of most reparation schemes reflects the continuing dominance of the retributive model; this, it is assumed, is what courts are about. Many practitioners are, it is true, attracted by the idea of making amends, but these same practitioners (or their predecessors) have traditionally been pre-occupied with diversion. This has been allowed to take precedence. As a result, reparation schemes in England and Wales offer little challenge to the fundamental assumptions upon which the criminal justice system operates. The fact that reparation is so clearly seen as a way of influencing prosecution and/or sentencing decisions means that it is inextricably bound up with the notion of the tariff. Reparation is viewed as something separate, which it is hoped may appease a state punishing system. It is thereby marginalised, as reflected in the supplicatory posture adopted by reparation schemes towards the police or court. Reparation is seen as extraneous to the main business of the court – something which might be allowed to become a factor in mitigation.

There is, as already acknowledged, an alternative view of the appropriate institutional arrangements for reparation – and one which might be thought in keeping with the diversion principle. This is that reparation be developed alongside, but independent of, the state's response to a breach of criminal law. Reparation, on this view, is an appropriate response to behaviour which can plausibly be regarded as arising from a *dispute*. Furthermore, dispute is a kind of *pre*-crime; crime is what happens when disputes are not settled and get out of hand (Launay 1985). On this thinking the legal system is a last resort for 'trouble' which cannot be resolved in other, more constructive ways (Marshall 1985, p. 49). Marshall argues that courts are all very well for making public declarations about what is or is not acceptable behaviour, but other mechanisms are required if 'trouble' is to be resolved. He makes passing reference to the possibility of incorporating reparation within criminal justice – what he calls 'civilising' the existing system – but he is mainly concerned with the search for alternatives.

It has to be said that the practice of reparation schemes in England and Wales does not come close to matching the rhetoric of this dispute resolution model. Some cases are diverted from prosecution, and a few offenders may even be 'diverted' from prison, but there is precious little evidence of private settlement. Indeed, this is not the object. As Nelken (1986) has observed, current diversion policies are not operated in such a way as to be consistent with this view of the genesis of crime. Cases are diverted largely on the basis of their being low on the tariff (first offenders; relatively minor transgressions) rather than because they may plausibly be re-classified in terms of dispute. So minor shoplifting from a large store is subject to 'mediation'; serious assault involving friends or acquaintances tends not to be. This suggests that reparation is accorded a subordinate position (subordinate, that is, to the primary goals of diversion and mitigation) even where its adherents claim to adopt a dispute-resolution model.

The lesson to be drawn from this is not that retributive and reparative principles cannot be reconciled (see Watson et al, 1989). It is rather that reparation, if it is to be attempted at all, must be seen as part of the justice process – as a way of achieving justice (or a contribution towards achieving justice), not as a mechanism which enables some offenders to *evade* justice. If priority if given to diversion, reparation schemes will not attract support. They will come to be regarded as a means whereby some offenders evade, not only retributive justice, but reparative justice as well.

Chapter 7

Neglected themes I
Negotiation and expiation

Few would dissent from the proposition that offenders should be rendered accountable for their actions – that, due regard having been taken of their social circumstances and any other mitigating factors, they should be required to take responsibility for what they have done. The expressions 'rendered accountable' and 'take responsibility' might be thought to have a punitive ring, but, as Howard Zehr points out (1985), this reflects the retributive ethos with which we are familiar and which is to be found within our criminal courts. Zehr argues that offenders need to be helped to understand the real human consequences of their actions; and, secondly, they need to be encouraged to do everything in their power to right the wrong which they have done. Through such actions they express repentance and, just as important, have the hope of forgiveness. In that sense making amends is as important to offenders as it is to victims; how else, Zehr asks, are they to put their pasts behind them?

It is beyond question that there is no serious attempt, within the criminal justice system as it stands, to pursue this objective. Admittedly the 1959 White Paper, *Penal Practice in a Changing Society*, did argue that 'the redemptive value of the punishment to the offender would be greater if it were made to include the realisation of the injury he had done to his victim as well as to the order of society and the need to make proper reparation for that injury', but prior to the mid 1980s there was no significant policy initiative. There were frequent references in the courts to offenders having to be held accountable for their actions, but 'accountability' was limited to the notion that when you do something wrong you must take your punishment (Zehr 1985; Braithwaite 1989). Zehr observes that the justice process not only fails to encourage offenders to understand what it is that they have done; it actively discourages such an understanding. Far from encouraging the offender to make amends, the process promotes anger, rationalisation, denial of responsibility, and a sense of powerlessness and dehumanisation, so that 'as with victims, the wound will fester and grow' (Zehr 1985).

Christie (1977) comes to a very similar conclusion. He describes the offender as 'a listener to a discussion – often a highly unintelligible one – of how much pain he ought to receive', rather than a participant in an enquiry into the nature of the offence and an exploration of how to make good the harm done. He is also denied the opportunity to explain himself to the victim, so losing the opportunity to seek or be offered forgiveness. This theme is echoed by Priestley and McGuire who contrast the emphasis given to establishing the offender's *responsibility* for the offence with the subsequent treatment of him as wholly *irresponsible* – an object upon whom pain and deprivation are to be visited in proportion to the harm done . . .

> the offence becomes a public property whose title can be redeemed only by symbolic repayments in a currency of loss and suffering to be undergone by the offender. Thus dispossessed, he feels absolved of all further interest in his 'case' and concerned only with enduring the deprivations imposed on him as a sentence of the court. This fundamental irresponsibility can only intensify the already poor picture of him or herself held by many an offender.
>
> (Priestley and McGuire 1985, p. 51)

It may be thought especially surprising that the theme of personal responsibility attracts so little interest given our Christian tradition. According to Thatcher (1991), Christianity provides a framework within which reparation, mediation and reconciliation are fundamental motifs. Despite growing secularisation (Chadwick 1975), we still regard ourselves as a Christian country, and yet an important strand of Christian thinking about the appropriate response to wrong-doing finds little or no expression within our criminal courts. Christian thought yields one non-retributive theory of punishment which is of special relevance – 'the symbolic theory' (Thatcher 1991). According to the symbolic theory, the punishment of an offender is intended to arrest or reverse his moral decline as manifested by the offence (Moberly 1978, p. 64). Punishment prospectively symbolises the moral end of the unreformed offender. It is also intended to make good the wrong (Thatcher 1991; Moberly

1978, p. 69). As Thatcher explains, mediation affords an opportunity for the offender to be confronted by the horror of innocent suffering and his responsibility for this. It could, therefore, be the means to avert his moral decline. For victims, mediation affords an opportunity to express forgiveness, thereby discharging the pain of innocent suffering.

The symbolic theory greatly enriches the 'justice as balance' formulation which traditionally underpins not only retributivism, but also most attempts to promote reparation. It places reparation in a *redemptive* context . . . 'the symbolic theory . . . transforms the aims of punishment so that they become the forestalling of the consequences of wrong-doing and the transformation of the wrong-doer' (Thatcher 1991). As Thatcher explains, to view punishment in these terms provides a new role for reparation under which equivalence is eclipsed by more important considerations. Reparation could provide the opportunity to transform the attitudes of both parties, something which conventional punishment does not even attempt. Mediation and reparation schemes, it might therefore be argued, give practical expression to the symbolic theory. This indeed is Thatcher's view. He suggests that 'a principal merit of mediation and reparation schemes is that they already present a working model of the symbolic theory of punishment without apparent knowledge of its philosophical and theological roots' (Thatcher 1991). He develops this point in order to argue that 'an explicit knowledge of the symbolic theory would help to clarify the thinking of those involved in operating the schemes . . . and provide a convincing framework for their interpretation' (ibid). Unfortunately, reparation in England and Wales is severely under-theorised. The case study material in Chapters 3 to 5 indicates that the failure to come to terms with reparation's various philosophical and theological roots, to which Thatcher alludes, has undermined the practice of the various schemes. As was noted in Chapter 6, this is largely focused upon the offender's interests in the far narrower sense of assisting him or her to avoid punishment.

It is interesting to observe that one society within which 'justice as balance' is less dominant, or so it would appear, is non-Christian Japan. According to Haley (1989), a 'leitmotif' of confession, repentance and absolution dominates each stage of law enforcement in Japan: 'From the initial police interrogation to the final judicial hearing on sentencing, the vast majority of those accused of criminal offences confess, display repentance, negotiate for their victims' pardon and submit to the mercy of the authorities. In return they are treated with extraordinary leniency; they gain at least the prospect of absolution by being dropped from the formal process altogether' (Haley 1989). Haley quotes Minoru Shikita, former director of the United Nations Asia and Far East Institute for the Prevention of Crime and Treatment of Offenders, as observing that:

> the police . . . need not refer all cases formally to the prosecution . . . provided the offences are minor property offences, the suspects have shown repentance, restitution has been made, and victims forgive the suspects.
>
> (Shikita 1982, p. 37)

Even in cases referred to public prosecutors, 'the police invariably recommend a lenient disposition if a suspect has shown sincere repentance about his or her alleged crime and the transgression . . . is not particularly serious' (ibid, p. 37). According to Haley, Japanese judges 'uniformly confirm that the defendant's acknowledgment of guilt, sincerity in displaying remorse, evidenced in part by compensation of the victim and the victim's forgiving response, are pivotal in their decision on whether to suspend sentence' (Haley 1989).

Whether such expressions of remorse are genuine, or whether, perhaps, the pressure towards public repentance generates resentment as much as contrition, is a matter which it is impossible at this distance to determine. One may suspect that confession, repentance, and absolution have become less evident as Japan has become more Westernised. That still leaves open the question of why these ideas, which have permeated Japanese culture for centuries, find so little expression in advanced Western societies with a Christian tradition. This, perhaps, reflects the complicated and contradictory nature of the Christian message in respect of punishment and wrong-doing. Some aspects of this message have been absorbed and acted upon; others are accorded no more than lip service. Mediation and reparation schemes in England and Wales offer an antidote to the harsh equalisation which is one part of the Christian message (and, arguably, the only part which is reflected in the practice of our criminal courts), but they fail to utilise another branch of Christian theology with which they might be expected to be in accord.

They also fail to utilise (or utilise in sporadic, half-hearted fashion) the most powerful psychological theory offered in explanation of the offender's capacity to perform (and go on performing) anti-social acts. This is Sykes and Matza's *techniques of neutralisation* (Sykes and Matza 1957). These authors argue that much delinquency is based on an unrecognised psychological defence to the commission of such acts, namely, a series of justifications which are seen as valid by the delinquent although not by society at large. Disapproval is 'neutralised' by a series of rationalisations. These permit the delinquent to have his cake and eat it in that he remains committed to some version of the dominant social norms, and yet is able to violate them. As Sykes and Matza put it, 'the delinquent represents not a radical opposition to law-abiding society but something more like an apologetic failure, often more sinned against than sinning in his own eyes' (ibid).

Sykes and Matza suggest that there are in fact five major techniques of neutralisation:

1. denial of responsibility ('I didn't mean it');
2. denial of injury ('I didn't really hurt anybody');
3. denial of the victim ('they had it coming to them');
4. condemnation of the condemners ('everybody's picking on me');
5. appeal to higher loyalties ('I didn't do it for myself').

These slogans, Sykes and Matza argue, function as defences for transgressions already committed and also prepare for the commission of further delinquent acts. The justifications are not invented by the offender; they are borrowed from the dominant normative system. It follows therefore that identifying these techniques of neutralisation does not merely provide us with one way of understanding delinquent behaviour; it also suggests a means whereby such behaviour might be challenged. The clue to this lies in the fact (as it is hypothesised) that the dominant normative system is not rejected in its entirety by the delinquent; it is merely struck a 'glancing blow', as Sykes and Matza put it. So offenders' justifications can be challenged and undermined by reference to standards which they themselves accept. This is occasionally reflected in the practice of UK reparation schemes, as in one or two instances which we observed at Coventry, but the under-theorised nature of mediation and reparation initiatives in England and Wales means that no scheme sets out consciously to challenge techniques of neutralisation.

The same cannot be said of Germany, where Messmer's work demonstrates the value of a properly theorised practice. This theoretical underpinning is provided by Sykes and Matza's neutralisation thesis, somewhat modified by Messmer who develops an alternative set of 'justifications'. These have particular relevance to the build-up to a fight/assault (the form of transgression with which Messmer is particularly concerned). He identifies four main types of justification:

1. The construction of competing versions of the conflict (who provoked whom etc);
2. The construction of competing norm concepts (alternative codes of honourable behaviour are advanced and certain conventional behaviour is denigrated as being dishonourable, e.g. failure to participate in a fair fight, reporting the matter to the police, etc);
3. The construction of doubts about the consequences of the offence (e.g. the assertion that compensation claims are inflated);
4. The construction of negative characterisations of the opposing party.

These justifications are employed not only to rationalise the behaviour in question, but also to achieve a favourable outcome to the subsequent negotiation. The negotiation itself therefore involves, first, the construction of favourable positions by the person accused of wrong-doing, and second, the breaking down of those positions. The process is one in which competing accounts are delivered; systems of justification are advanced; and those same justifications are countered and undermined. As Messmer puts it: 'Justifications which are meant to neutralise the consequences of an offence must themselves be neutralised.' In the course of the negotiation certain propositions or perspectives have to be abandoned in the face of contradictory evidence. At the same time, additional grievances may be identified so that, for example, one originating cause (say, of a fight) may be elaborated into a whole system of accusations. This means that the course of the negotiation is unpredictable. It is not possible to determine in advance which element of justification will most readily be broken down and will therefore provide the basis for a successful negotiation.

For this kind of negotiation to succeed it is essential that the parties confront one another directly. These non-congruent perspectives cannot be challenged effectively at second hand; indeed, some of these viewpoints may not be relayed to third parties – they will only emerge in the course of face to face negotiation. The mediator assists the process by breaking down the vicious circle of accusation followed by heightened resistance and denial. Typically, the offender's justifications are not rejected out of hand, but contradictory perspectives are asserted as being equally valid. In this way the offender may gain insight into the impact of his behaviour on others so that their perspective – initially at odds with his own – may be acknowledged and granted validity. The procedures governing the negotiation have to be flexible in order that the parties to the conflict may raise all the issues which they consider relevant. This perhaps presents the most obvious contrast with the way in which the same behaviour (say, an assault) would be dealt with in a court.

The reparation schemes which we observed (and I believe their approach reflects that of virtually all schemes in England and Wales) did not display the procedural flexibility which Messmer argues is essential if the parties are to be permitted to raise all those issues which they deem to be important. Nor was there any attempt at the kind of direct confrontation between victim and offender which, Messmer suggests, is necessary in order for the offender's self-justificatory view of events to be undermined. In some cases, as we have seen, the 'reparation' undertaken was so perfunctory that it could only be understood as a kind of ritual obeisance to a retributive system. The remedial actions performed by the offender were assigned a reparative label but were devoid of reparative content. At other centres, notably Coventry, the offender was not given such an easy ride, but this was at the hands of *the mediator*; the encounter between victim and offender was carefully constructed so as to be devoid of any element of challenge, confrontation, or indeed of negotiation. An encounter which both sides might have found difficult and memorable was played out according to rules which robbed it of most of its meaning but rendered it *safe* (that is to say, unchallenging). It was safe for the offender, safe for the victim, and, above all, safe for the mediator.

This is not to deny that the Coventry scheme, in particular, had therapeutic objectives. The director of the project, especially, was committed to changing offender attitudes. To this end she arranged repeated interviews with offenders in the course of which she would attempt to test their motivation. It seemed to us, as researchers, that this had little to do with reparation; we would rather describe it as an imaginative form of probation work, using *the image* of the victim in an attempt to promote a re-think. The offender's eventual encounter with the victim may have been nerve-racking in prospect, but when it eventually arrived it was invariably undemanding in its content. The level of demand placed on the offender *prior* to meeting the victim was a deliberate attempt, so it seemed to us, to raise anxiety. This can be explained as a necessary counter-balance to the problem of offender inducement, this being a major difficulty for the schemes which we observed. Because the forms of reparation fostered in England and Wales are almost invariably non-material and, furthermore, undertaken in the shadow of a pending or threatened court appearance, 'impure motives' are always going to be a problem. One way to overcome this, as in the mediations studied by Messmer, is through a (necessarily painful) process of negotiation and re-evaluation, involving both parties to the original incident. At Coventry, they tried to achieve the same end by making offenders *think about* their victims. The mediators appeared to have limited faith that exposure to victim anger and distress would in itself promote the desired attitude change. They therefore tended to rely heavily on their own efforts in face to face discussion with the offender, held in advance of any meeting with the victim.

In all three schemes which we observed it appeared that the mediators were seeking to promote an exchange which was predictable – where the ground had already been laid. When a meeting between victim and offender did then take place there was an air of unease and of 'performance' about the encounter, with one or both parties appearing embarrassed and unsure as to what was expected of them. The uncertainty manifested on these occasions led us to ask: whose was the agenda? and, whence the motivation? Most victims did not manifest a strong desire to meet the offender in their case. They often gave the impression that they would be quite happy to forget the whole thing. There was no sense of the two sides being involved in an on-going dispute. Therein, I believe, lies much of the problem. People who are aggrieved, or who are in dispute, know what they want to say to one another. But where there is no issue, or the issue died a death some months before, the parties may well need some coaching and the exchanges may be marked by embarrassed, forced politeness, with both sides seeking to meet the mediator's expectations.

There is, I should acknowledge, an alternative view. Tony Marshall, co-ordinator of the various researches into Home Office sponsored reparation schemes, has claimed that:

> The best results usually followed careful preparation of both parties for mediation. An encounter between a victim and an offender is unlikely to be a situation either party is familiar with or able to use to greatest effect without guidance . . . Sometimes

the victim will need a great deal of help to deal with the emotional problems arising from the crime, but offenders are often
lacking the social skills that would enable them to present themselves convincingly and agreeably and may therefore require quite
a lot of preparation too. Those offenders who still fail to realise
the full extent of their personal responsibility may also be
prepared for the process of facing up to themselves and their
accountability that the meeting with the victim should complete.

(Marshall 1988)

Marshall's observations merit careful scrutiny because they are all too
revealing of the theoretical void which lay behind reparation initiatives in England and Wales. Why should offenders be trained to
present themselves convincingly and agreeably? Is there an argument, in that case, for the employment of a drama coach? What
happened to the insight – for which there *is* research evidence – that
offenders find it difficult to sustain their rationalisations when confronted by victims of their own or similar crimes, to whom they
accord 'high face validity' (Launay 1985)? Why, in the practice of
even the more convincing UK schemes, such as Coventry, is there a
continued preference for the probation model in which offender and
practitioner spend a great deal of time closeted together, with no
victim in sight? No convincing psychological explanation is offered
as to why preparatory meetings with the mediator should promote
attitude change. The assertion that 'the best results' were achieved
thereby is entirely unsubstantiated.

I would conclude from this that reparation schemes in England
and Wales were not principally concerned to resolve disputes, or to
promote offender attitude change. If they had been they would have
engaged in a much more demanding practice, with the contradictory
accounts of victim and offender providing the focal point. The only
negotiation which we observed was that between the mediator and
victim or offender *separately* – never together. That is not to say that
nothing of value emerged from the victim/offender meetings which
we observed – see, for example, the Michael Morley case at Totton
– but all too often the dominant impression was that of a performance in which two inexperienced actors struggled with unfamiliar
lines for the benefit of an unseen audience. That audience comprised
either the Juvenile Liaison Bureau or the court; the former would
already have delivered their verdict (thumbs up), whilst the latter
would do so in a few weeks' time.

Chapter 8

Neglected themes II
The victim interest

There have been a number of imaginative accounts of the predicament of crime victims, each of them identifying the neglect which victims suffer at the hands of a criminal justice apparatus whose ostensible purpose is to respond to the injury which they have suffered (see, for example, Christie 1977; Priestley and McGuire 1985; Zehr 1990). Priestley and McGuire describe the way in which

> once an offence has been committed, the momentum of the criminal justice machine carries it onward towards the fulfilment of a single aim: the apprehension, scrutiny, and processing of the offender. The other party involved in the offence – the victim – is almost entirely absent from the scene. Accustomed as we are to this state of affairs, it is difficult even to perceive how unnatural it is. Our whole conception of what it means to break the law and what should happen afterwards is cast in terms of it; and its influence on what we do with offenders, and thereby on their subsequent behaviour, must be both pervasive and profound.
>
> (Priestley and McGuire 1985, p. 206)

Christie likewise focuses upon this failure to involve the victim in the resolution of his own case. His theme is one of lost opportunity. Crime is an expression of conflict – and conflict, in Christie's eyes, is central to our role as citizens. It ought therefore to generate activity on the part of those directly involved. But the victim is denied this opportunity because the task of responding to crime is monopolised by professionals:

> [The victim] has lost participation in his own case. It is the Crown that comes into the spotlight, not the victim. It is the Crown that describes the losses, not the victim. It is the Crown that appears in

the newspaper, very seldom the victim. It is the Crown that gets a chance to talk to the offender, and neither the Crown nor the offender are particularly interested in carrying on that conversation. The prosecutor is fed-up long since. The victim would not have been. He might have been scared to death, panic-stricken, or furious. But he would not have been un-involved. It would have been one of the important days in his life. Something that belonged to him has been taken away from that victim.

(Christie 1977)

There is a tendency, these days, to treat Christie's vision with condescension, assuming it to represent an over-romanticised vision of tribal justice which could never be applied to our society of strangers. But what Christie has to say about the plight of victims can be confirmed by stepping inside any criminal court. The proceedings truly are bizarre in their rigidity, their narrow focus, and in denying a voice to those who should be the key participants. The most dramatic and tragic human events are reduced to a level of stunning banality and tedium.

VICTIM NEEDS

The last decade has seen a modest amount of government attention paid to the needs of crime victims, while victims have become a reputable, albeit still minor focus of criminological interest (see, in particular, Shapland et al, 1985; Mawby and Gill 1987; Maguire and Corbett 1987; Maguire and Pointing 1988; Walklate 1989; and Rock 1990). We now know something about how victims feel in the aftermath of crime, principally through the work of Shapland and her colleagues (1985) and through a smaller study by O'Brien (1986). For example, the number of victims and offenders who had a prior personal relationship is perhaps greater than was previously thought. O'Brien found that almost a quarter of her (admittedly modest) sample of victims knew the offender well, he/she being a relative or close associate, whilst a further quarter knew the offender slightly, or saw him/her in the neighbourhood.

The Shapland and O'Brien studies are also interesting on the question of whether victims had any desire to meet the offender again, perhaps to confront him with the consequences of his action and to seek an explanation. Fifteen per cent of the victims in

Shapland's study said that they would like to meet the offender again, while 34 per cent of O'Brien's (much smaller) sample said the same. O'Brien found that victims who had the most problems, or who were most upset, were least likely to want such a meeting; and in general victims did not wish to meet the offender if they had previously formed a poor view of his character. We are deprived of further insight into victims' response by the untimely death of Ann Garton, who had been monitoring the Leeds Reparation Scheme. Her work revealed the extent of victims' anger in the aftermath of an offence, a topic which would have been the subject of her Ph.D. thesis. In her interim report Garton observed that:

> While some victims are emotionally upset, virtually all are angry; they have frequently been deterred from physical retaliation against the offender only by the fear of the legal consequences and it is the presence of anger which invariably makes victims react negatively to the prospect of a meeting with their offender. This is a factor which has been identified on a practical level by mediators and a significant part of their task is to urge victims of the value of 'telling offenders what you think of them' i.e. to divert physical anger into verbal anger.
>
> (Garton 1986, 4:2)

One feature of most of the discussion of victim need (and, as I shall argue, a serious misrepresentation) is the contention that victims are comparatively uninterested in material compensation. Shapland identifies the strongest theme in her interviews as being victims' 'wish for respect and appreciation' (Shapland 1984). Whilst noting that between 57 per cent and 64 per cent of the victims in her sample would have welcomed financial compensation, she reports that 'the most striking result . . . is the persistence and consistency of the prevalence of physical, social and psychological effects over time, compared to the low level and decrease over time of financial loss' (Shapland 1984).

According to Shapland, such compensation as is paid 'appears to be on a different basis to that wanted by victims'. Compensation payments were regarded as important because of the acknowledgement thereby given to the victim within the criminal justice system . . .

> Even the element of payment in proportion to suffering and loss was subordinated to this symbolic function . . . It was not the

actual receipt of the money that was important, but the judgement which that award represented about the suffering and position of the victim.

(Shapland 1984)

Shapland's main point is that victims are not unduly punitive in seeking full compensation from impecunious offenders, but her findings have been interpreted as an indication that victims are not bothered about material loss, being mainly concerned that they be 'recognised' by the court (such recognition, it is implied, being independent of any order for compensation). This image of the non-punitive, non-materialistic victim may have been useful in countering an earlier mythology, but there is little doubt that it too is a myth – and a myth which has served to bolster forms of reparation which are grossly neglectful of the victim interest. Victims may well have 'unanswered questions' (Reeves 1984), but they would also like cheques. As it is, we find that a selective version of Shapland's findings is advanced by reparation schemes in defence of their circumscribed, pre-determined, and offender-orientated practice. This is also the tenor of the Home Office report on UK reparation schemes, with the authors citing Shapland's research in support of the proposition that 'the needs of victims are as often emotional as practical, and the former may be more important and almost certainly longer-lasting' (Marshall and Merry 1990).

THE CASE FOR COMPENSATION

The principle of compensation by offenders to victims who have suffered loss or injury through crime was introduced in 1973. This was extended by the Criminal Justice Act 1982 which provided that a compensation order could be employed as a sentence in its own right and that it should take precedence over a fine. Further encouragement was given to compensation when, in 1988, the government introduced a requirement that courts give their reasons for *not* awarding compensation in circumstances where the victim was eligible. These various attempts to promote compensation indicate that successive governments have been committed to the idea, even if the practice of courts remains equivocal.

The available research evidence suggests that crime victims endorse the principle that financial compensation should form one element within criminal proceedings. Of Shapland's group of 217 victims, 74 (34 per cent) had actually applied for compensation, while 57 per cent said that they would definitely have liked compensation, with a further 7 per cent unsure (Shapland 1984). The main reasons for *not* seeking compensation were the victim's acceptance that the offence was trivial, or that there were no specific expenses arising from it. Vennard's research, quoted by Shapland, leaves one in no doubt that the great majority of victims who suffered material loss would indeed welcome compensation (Vennard 1976). Shapland's summary of the weight of evidence is instructive in that it is clearly at odds with the message distilled from her work by apologists for the present reparation practice in this country:

> This almost unquestioning acceptance of the appropriateness of the principle of compensation from offenders, its place in the criminal justice system and, particularly, the preference for it amongst those who received such orders is striking. It contrasts vividly with the doubts of legal commentators.
>
> (Shapland 1984, p. 140)

That compensation is desired by victims does not mean, of course, that offenders have the means to pay (or to pay very much). Furthermore, less than 30 per cent of property offences lead to an arrest, while even those cases in which an arrest is made may not lead to prosecution; or the offender may be prosecuted but not convicted; or he may be convicted and sent to prison. One can see, therefore, that compensation ordered through the criminal courts can assist only a minority of victims (Campbell 1984), while such payments as are made may cover a mere fraction of the loss, and be long delayed (Reeves 1984). It is for this reason that the 'welfare' model of compensation (Campbell 1984), as reflected in the Criminal Injuries Compensation Board, offers a more realistic hope of compensation for most victims – provided, that is, that they fall within the scope of the scheme. Successive UK governments have accepted the potentially heavy financial obligation that this entails, although such provision is limited to physical injury, it being left to private insurance to cover material loss. The CICB has been in operation for twenty-five years and was recently put on a statutory basis, conferring a right to compensation upon those who satisfy certain conditions. In 1988 the Board paid out £52 million to 30,000 claimants, while in 1989 the chairman, Lord Carlisle, announced that the Board was then dealing with 1,000 new claimants a week and had a backlog of over 85,000 cases (*The Observer*, 9/7/89).

Whilst there is little likelihood, in the majority of cases of injury or loss, that payment by the offender will provide adequate compensation for victims, this is no reason to deny the centrality of financial compensation to the justice process. Campbell (1984) argues very convincingly that reparation should be regarded as part of punishment (see also Watson et al, 1989). It is not merely a 'welfare' concept designed to assist victims, nor a therapeutic measure aimed at offenders. Instead, as Campbell puts it, the objective of reparation should be:

> to remedy the injustice which crime creates between offender and victim. Reparation may therefore be a goal to be striven for even if it cannot be fully attained, just as prevention and deterrence are penal objectives which can be only partly realised, but are not therefore unimportant.
>
> (Campbell 1984)

To regard compensation as part of punishment is an important conceptual shift. It allows that reparation be brought within the halls of justice, rather than being permitted a status equivalent only to that of a beggar at the gate. It gives expression to our common understanding (abandoned as we cross the threshold of the courtroom) that the individual victim, as well as 'the fabric of society', has been damaged by the offender's activities. Indeed, it is inevitable that the victim's loss is more immediate and more grievous (Campbell 1984); what kind of justice process is it that can ignore this fundamental fact?

REPARATION AND VICTIMS: THE OFFICIAL VIEW

Early government presentation of compensation and reparation initiatives stressed the victim interest. Rock (1990) demonstrates the way in which criminal injuries compensation, crime surveys, victim support, and reparation were presented as elements within a single package. They were all part of the Home Office's 'victim policy'. The Report of the Parliamentary All-Party Penal Affairs Group (1984) treated criminal injuries compensation, reparation, and victim support as a single issue. So did the 1984 Report of the Home Affairs Select Committee. The Home Office's statement of strategic objectives, *Criminal Justice: A Working Paper* (Home Office 1986a), grouped police reform, financial compensation by offenders, criminal injuries compensation, and victim support schemes under

the single heading 'Helping the Victim'. When it came to the
reparation initiatives taken in the mid 1980s, the Home Office
claimed in its press release heralding *Reparation: A Discussion
Document* (Home Office 1986), that the purpose of reparation, in
addition to enabling the offender to realise the full consequences of
what he had done, was 'to give reassurance and practical help to the
victim'.

In fact, the Home Office vision, as Rock well describes, was
directed *not* at the victim interest, but towards 'new, useful, and
efficient sanctions for a changing criminal justice system in a time of
high unemployment' (Rock 1990, p. 296). The Home Office intention at that time was to introduce a new court sentence – an
alternative disposal for low tariff offenders. Rock observes that 'reparation was often only rather obliquely directed at victims . . . There
was no talk of victims in many of the discussions about the new
reparation order and some involved officials said that it was "not
likely to bring benefits for victims"' (1990, p. 299). He concludes
that '(d)oing things to and for victims was always considered to be an
oblique way of confronting the penal crisis' (ibid, p. 366). This was
also the view taken by Helen Reeves, then Director of the National
Association of Victim Support Schemes. She observed of the All-
Party Penal Affairs publication, *A New Deal for Victims* (1984):
'they're all penal reformers and they're really enthusiastic about
finding alternatives to traditional penalties. To be frank, that's what
it's all about' (quoted in Rock 1990, p. 366).

There is some evidence that this same gap between rhetoric and
reality characterised North American initiatives. For example, Rock
describes how, in Ontario, victim–offender reconciliation 'was to be
the predominant theme in the Ministry's work with victims' – an
aspiration somewhat at odds with developments on the ground. Just
as in Britain, North American initiatives were focused primarily on
the offender . . .

> the intellectual and practical origins of restitution are . . . found in
> the innovative wing of American corrections, not in the victim
> movement . . . the majority of restitution programmes rarely
> concern themselves very much with making victims whole or
> attending to their needs, desires, or rights.
> (Hofrichter 1980, quoted in Rock 1990, p. 283)

The fact that, in reality, reparation schemes in England and Wales
were primarily interested in diversion, mitigation and offender

education did not stop an alliance developing between reparation practitioners (and enthusiasts generally) and the National Association of Victim Support Schemes. NAVSS became, as Rock describes, 'the reluctant, ambivalent mid-wife of reparation schemes', responding to queries, organising conferences, and doing much of the spade-work leading to the creation of FIRM (Forum for Initiatives in Reparation and Mediation). The Director of NAVSS recalls how 'Practitioners such as probation officers and lawyers appeared to accept without question that reparation was a victim service and Victims Support was congratulated on the amount of attention it was now receiving' (Reeves 1989).

This presentation of reparation as a victim service (in part, at least) was perpetuated by FIRM and by the schemes themselves. At a Conference at the University of Kent in March 1986, Tony Marshall, by then Director of FIRM, observed that 'it is up to all of us to initiate the necessary contacts and to demonstrate that mediation benefits the victim first, above all else.'

Press reporting, which was markedly enthusiastic for a time, also dwelt upon the benefits which victims might derive from the work of reparation schemes. For example, one laudatory account of the Totton scheme quoted the scheme's co-ordinator as follows:

> For the first time the victim is able to participate in the criminal justice process. Up until now victims have been excluded and have had nowhere to express their own feelings. Very often the only way they have learnt of the fate of the offender is through the local paper. No one has bothered to tell them. Mediation helps to resolve the feelings of the victims and gives them a chance to express how they feel on neutral ground within the community.
> (*The Independent*, 28.9.86)

VICTIMS IN THE SERVICE OF OFFENDERS

Our observation of reparation schemes in England and Wales convinced us that, despite the above claims, the term 'reparation' is applied to offender actions in the aftermath of crime which make little if any contribution to remedying the harm done to the victim. It is applied to letters written at the virtual dictation of a probation officer; to material reparation which is merely 'symbolic'; to an expressed willingness to *meet* the victim; and to muttered apology offered in the shadow of a pending (or threatened) court appearance. Thus, many UK schemes, interested primarily in diversion or mitigation, have manipulated the reparation concept to the point where it offers victims little beyond the possibility of serving the interests of 'their' offender (Davis et al, 1988). These schemes are mis-described in that their principal objective is not acknowledged. Diversion from prosecution or mitigation of the court's penalty cannot of themselves make good the harm done, so schemes having this as their *main* aim are better not described as reparation schemes: they are primarily concerned to achieve disposals least restrictive of the rights of offenders. Diversion from prosecution or mitigation of penalty may of course be justified on the basis of reparation made. Conscious of this, some schemes encourage offender actions which might plausibly be thought to contain a reparative element, but their main purpose remain that of advancing the case for diversion or mitigation. I would argue that the case for diversion (which, in many instances, is compelling) ought to be made on the grounds of labelling and contamination, rather than on the basis of 'reparation' which may be devoid of reparative content.

One consequence of the present uncomfortable relationship between reparation and the courts is that magistrates have come to regard reparation as an exercise undertaken primarily for the benefit of the offender. One magistrate whom we interviewed referred to the suspicion with which many of his fellows regarded the reparation concept. He illustrated this with reference to a colleague on the bench who had had her house burgled five times: he doubted whether she would want to meet 'her' burglars; *she had been too distressed by the experience to want to make any contribution to their welfare.* Given this view of reparation, one can understand concern about the possible pressure which may be brought to bear on victims by reparation schemes. It is all too easy to forget that reparation, on a perfectly natural construction, is primarily *for* victims. But the practice developed by some offender-orientated schemes, with staff who are interested in offender attitude change and, above all, in reducing the penalty imposed by a court, has almost no vestige of reparation discernible within it. From the victim's point of view, this is neither retributive justice nor reparative justice; it is no kind of justice at all.

Predictably, the mitigatory potential of reparation has been spotted by defence solicitors. We observed a case in Coventry magistrates court where the defence solicitor made great play of the benefit which the victim had derived from a meeting with the offender. But the victim was not present in court and it seemed clear that the reparation made in this case had really been for the benefit of the offender. The victim, unbeknown to herself, was being hauled into the mitigation process.

But the *main* reason to suppose that reparation is regarded principally as a means of deflecting or appeasing a retributive system is the fact that selection of cases for reparation is made entirely upon offender-based criteria, with the victim not even being consulted (Reeves 1989). This reflects the exclusive offender focus of the criminal justice system as a whole (offenders may not welcome this attention; and I am not suggesting that it is benevolent in its effects; merely that they are the recipients of it). Despite the rhetoric, reparation schemes go along with this exclusive offender focus rather than challenging it. The offender is the focus for the scheme, just as the offender is the focus for the court. One can see this in Coventry, for example, where the starting point for the mediator is a series of interviews with the offender in order to establish appropriate attitude. These meetings are held before the victims have been asked whether they are interested in reparation, and before they have been asked what form they would like that reparation (if any) to take.

The cases selected for reparation reflect the diversionary and mitigatory objectives; with a few exceptions, such as the Michael Morley case in Totton, most schemes gear their efforts towards low tariff offences and, one might say, low tariff offenders. Sometimes, as Young reports in relation to the Wolverhampton scheme, the victim had forgotten all about the offence by the time that the reparation proposal was put to him or her. Slightly comically, this phenomenon of the forgetful victim has been ascribed to a problem of timing (Marshall 1986). Marshall alludes to the difficulty presented by victims who are 'either too angry or not angry enough' at the time the mediation proposal is put. He suggests that 'it would be preferable for schemes to be able to adjust the timing of a meeting to the psychodynamic career of the victim . . . a scheme should obtain referrals at as early a stage as possible in order to catch those parties whose upset is likely to be short-lived'. The problem, it need hardly be said, is not merely one of timing; viewed from the victim perspective, current reparation practice raises fundamental questions of relevance. This is despite the fact that many victims, whether they have suffered property offences or offences of violence, would indeed welcome an opportunity to confront the offender with the consequences of his actions and, as it may be, to negotiate some material recompense.

THE NEGLECT OF MATERIAL REPARATION

The reparation schemes which we studied were uninterested in material reparation. It has been suggested that the practice of UK schemes provides 'one of the first practical tests, albeit rudimentary and unsystematic, [of a restitution-based justice process]' (Marshall and Merry 1990). Unfortunately, that is not the case. The various schemes differed from one another in important respects, but one feature which they had in common was their neglect of restitution. The Coventry scheme, also researched by Richard Young, may be regarded as typical in this respect. The Coventry mediators were interested in offender attitude change and mitigation; they did not, in our experience, broach the topic of restitution. As Young points out, if victims declined to meet their offender they might be asked if they would accept a written apology; but they would not be asked if they were interested in financial compensation (Young 1987a).

Most UK schemes do not acknowledge that the failure to institute restitution arises from their own lack of interest in this form of reparation; they say it is because *victims* are not interested. But, as Young points out, whereas responsibility for the paucity of restitution agreements is attributed to the victim, 'nothing is said of the possible role the scheme has played in moulding those wishes . . . it is clear that a mediator may have a significant degree of control over both the process of mediation and its outcome' (Young 1987a). As is apparent from Chapter 10, and revealed also in the writings of Howard Zehr, the practice amongst US reparation schemes is quite different. Zehr explains the American thinking (and practice) as follows:

> Reparation (by which he means 'restitution') is not the primary goal, but it is often an important part of the process. Victims usually participate in the first place on the understanding that reparation may be possible, even if afterwards they come to value other aspects of the mediation more. Reparation is both an important symbol and a concrete recognition of the offender's remorse and obligations. Reparation does not have to constitute complete repayment to be these things. Is this emphasis just a matter of American materialism? I don't think it is wholly so. The victim does have certain rights to restitution and the offender corresponding obligations, and these must not be denied.
>
> (Zehr 1988)

In the USA they term their reparation schemes 'Victim/Offender Reconciliation Programs' (VORPs), but it is understood that reconciliation will, in most instances, require an element of restitution. The UK schemes likewise aspire towards reconciliation, but the mediators tend to believe that this can be achieved without any attempt to make good the material loss. Marshall suggests that the different practices may be explained by the fact that victims in this country have alternative sources of compensation (Marshall 1986), but this is hardly a plausible explanation. Few victims in the cases we observed were likely to be compensated through the courts (and none by means of the CICB). The real reason for the difference in practice between the two countries is that the staff of UK reparation schemes are either not interested in or are positively uncomfortable at the thought of helping to negotiate restitution. This is consistent with habits of thought developed in the course of their earlier probation practice – they are interested in lightening the load on offenders, not, as it may appear, in increasing it. Furthermore, there is no certainty that a compensation agreement would serve to mitigate more effectively than would, say, a willingness to meet and apologise. This clear offender orientation is inevitable given that most reparation schemes in England and Wales have developed under the aegis of the probation service. But this may produce a considerable distortion of the reparation concept (Zehr 1986).

Young's interviews with victims whose cases had been referred to the Coventry scheme suggest that the most disappointed – and therefore the most critical – were those who had sought an element of material reparation (Young 1987a). Young suggests that the ideal victim from the scheme's point of view would have suffered in a personal capacity; would be experiencing continuing feelings of anger or insecurity; would be alienated by his/her lack of involvement in the justice process; and would have had a prior personal relationship with the offender that was in need of repair. But in most cases there was in fact no such relationship and the main impact of the offence upon the victim lay in the financial loss and inconvenience . . . 'the offence was regarded as annoying rather than as a traumatic experience' (ibid). So victims might be interested in material reparation, but because the mediators were preoccupied with resolution through talking (and with symbolic gestures of reconciliation), victims' preference for getting their money back might remain unvoiced and unrecognised.

Both Young at Coventry and Ann Garton who researched the Leeds scheme suggest that material reparation assumed symbolic as well as practical significance for victims. Had it existed, it would have been the one element in the whole process which was manifestly geared to their interest rather than to that of the offender (Young 1987a; Garton 1986). Young and Garton, independently of one another, suggest that this preoccupation with mitigating sentence, coupled with the failure to confront the issue of material reparation, led victims to regard the mediators' efforts with scepticism. To ignore restitution might not have been so bad in itself, but to do this whilst clearly intending that such reparation as was performed should serve to mitigate gave rise to very considerable dissatisfaction on the part of some victims. They felt they were being used.

There has been a concerted attempt – led by Tony Marshall, former Director of FIRM and co-ordinator of Home Office research on reparation – to play down the importance of restitution. For example, Marshall asserts that:

> A stress on material negotiations about the appropriate quantum for reparation may be seen as sullying the enlightening exchange of views that the more successful mediation meetings can provoke . . . the calculating and commercial nature of negotiating compensation may well inhibit the kind of exchange that could produce catharsis and satisfactory mutual understanding . . . disagreements over the extent of damage or what was stolen and its value might be far from easy for the mediator to manage, apart from any effect such wrangling might have on the newly-formed and fragile relationship between the two.
>
> (Marshall and Merry 1990)

Marshall claims that the evidence from the Home Office sponsored reparation research supports his contention that victims are uninterested in restitution and/or that mediation is an inappropriate vehicle through which to negotiate money:

> One of the findings of this research is that the importance of material reparation for victims has been over-stressed in the past . . . negotiations about material quanta (compensation to be paid, hours to be worked) tended to be divisive and disruptive to a mediation process that was intended to bring the parties closer in terms of understanding and personal communication. Neither

mediators nor parties seemed to find it easy to pass from the emotionally-charged exchange of explanations, apology and for-giveness to an anti-climactic discussion of material things.

(Marshall 1986)

The impression one gets from the research is that victims would find it inappropriate to enter into personal negotiations in this way and would rather leave it to the court.

(Marshall and Merry 1990)

Marshall's role as research co-ordinator has led him to act as mouth-piece for UK reparation research as a whole, but his observations are markedly at odds with the evidence presented by all the more rigorous studies which have been exposed to public view. While it is a truism to say that one cannot have 'pure' research, uncontaminated by the researcher's own values and prior assumptions, there must be a willingness to take on board contradictory or perplexing material and to incorporate this into one's theorising. The compilation of UK research findings prepared by Marshall and Merry (1990) reflects Marshall's prior conception of what mediation and reparation should be about – and his is a peculiarly sentimental vision. Agreed, restitu-tion is not possible in every case; and *complete* restitution may be possible in very few cases; but to the extent that restitution is feasible, but remains undone, it is difficult to see how an apology could be thought sincere, or reconciliation achieved.

VICTIMS' WILLINGNESS TO ENGAGE IN MEDIATION

There was one unexpected finding of this research . . . It would seem that many – both academics and practitioners – have done victims the discredit of regarding them as motivated solely by personal gain. It seems that many have imagined that victims might go away with great glee with a wad of banknotes in their hands, or the promise of someone to slave in their garden. It is reassuring to find that the great majority of victims involved in these schemes were not so grasping, and indeed that they even seemed to feel rather guilty about taking something from the offender that by the usual norms of justice might have been seen as owing to them by right. The most frequent motive evidenced by those taking part in the schemes was, by contrast, *a desire to help*, a feeling of social concern.

(Marshall and Merry 1990)

What is clear . . . is the fact that victims rarely spontaneously agree
to mediation; persuasion is an integral part of mediator training.

(Garton 1986)

While the above extracts offer contrasting assessments of victims'
attitude to mediation, they are not *entirely* contradictory, although
the emphasis is very different. If schemes' definition of success is,
first, to secure a meeting, and second, to influence the sentence of
the court, a necessary pre-condition is that they get the victim to
engage in the process. This means that victims are likely to feel a
pressure: (a) to accept the offer of mediation; and (b) to agree to
some form of 'reparation' – if only because they do not want to feel
responsible for the offender being sent to prison. Some mediators,
indeed, regarded it as rather unreasonable of victims not to be
prepared to meet 'their' offender. At Leeds, for example, whilst it
was accepted that some victims were too upset to be asked to do this,
if victims were unwilling to take part because they were too angry,
or they wanted to wash their hands of the whole affair, they were
regarded as 'meanies'.

The means by which schemes sought to achieve higher levels of
victim participation are familiar to researchers faced with the problem of achieving a high interview success rate. At both Leeds and
Rochdale we were told that the mediator might make a return visit
in cases where the victim was initially reluctant to take part. When
the Leeds scheme first started, the mediators would see the offender
first, then the victim. However, two years later . . . 'we now see the
victim first and say we will be seeing the offender and "can I come
back and tell you about him?" This gives a second bite to the cherry'.
This is consistent with Ann Garton's finding that a refusal by either
party (most usually the victim) was seen as a failure . . . 'Although in
training there is a stress on the voluntary nature of the process and an
awareness of the undesirability of pressure, mediators are inclined to
value "persistence"' (Garton 1986).

One can detect here the seeds of a moral dilemma for mediators
in that they may not find it politic to confess their mitigatory
objective to victims. The co-ordinator of the Leeds scheme told us
that his staff asked victims quite explicitly whether they would be
prepared to help the offender. As one member of their management
committee put it, they approached victims on the basis that 'prison
doesn't work; we want the offender to change; can you help us?'
Garton, on the other hand, observed that the Leeds mediators

experienced considerable difficulty in giving victims an honest account of the scheme's objectives. This was because many victims would not have been in sympathy with the scheme's main aim of diverting the offender from a custodial sentence. She went so far as to suggest that 'the variable success of mediators in achieving victim co-operation . . . may reflect the extent to which they explain their task' (Garton 1986).

Arguably, the problem of victim coercion only arises because the probation service has manipulated the reparation concept to the point where it offers victims little, if anything, beyond the possibility of serving the interests of the offender. It should be acknowledged, however, that many victims agree to participate despite realising full well that any meeting will be geared primarily to the offender interest. In some instances their perception of the offender is not very different from that of the mediators, that is, as a vulnerable, disadvantaged youngster, in need of a helping hand. Exeter, for example, informed us that some corporate victims regarded their participation as a form of public service; there was even a standing arrangement with some large stores that the store would respond to offenders' letters in shoplifting cases. So it is not my contention that victims are to any significant extent being dragooned into accepting reparation. By and large they enter into these arrangements with their eyes open. But this does not alter the fact that reparation is largely being promoted with the offender's interest in mind. Victims therefore need to be mature, socially responsible citizens, interested in the welfare of 'their' offender. Many victims, of course, do not think like this and some crimes hardly permit a charitable reaction. But Marshall is right to the extent that many victims are quite tolerant of youthful transgression. However, our reaction to this should not simply be to breathe a collective sigh of relief; it should be another cause for regret – regret that victim compassion and decency, just as much as victim suffering, are at present excluded from those forums (either courts or social work offices) within which we determine the fate of offenders.

SYMBOLISM, FORGIVENESS, JUSTICE, AND VICTIMOLOGY

Philip Priestley (1977) has argued that it is inappropriate to view prisons and judicial processes as if they were rational responses to offending behaviour; this is because courts and prisons serve primarily *symbolic* purposes (including the definition of behavioural boundaries; the articulation of a secular account of good and evil; and the promotion of social solidarity and cohesion). If any proposal reform measure is to succeed, Priestley avers, it has to address the symbolic function of those punishments which it is intended to replace. He goes on to suggest that the relationship between offenders and their victims offers one fertile ground for alternative symbolic activity.

This is indeed a striking assessment, delivered well in advance of any institutional steps to promote reparation. It is striking because it contains within it important clues as to why reparation in England and Wales attracted such enthusiastic support, and why, in the end, it proved such a frustrating failure. Reparation has indeed gone down the 'symbolic' route – the treatment of victims reveals that to be the case. But courts and prisons are hugely powerful symbols, whilst the forms of reparation which we observed were all too obviously designed to appease a punishing system. Paradoxically, they lacked symbolic power because they were conceived from the outset as symbols. This is surely not what Priestley meant. You cannot have symbolism without first having substance; sending someone to prison is not just a matter of 'show' – he's locked up. But reparation schemes, by and large, put their faith in appearances. Sadly for them, this was never sufficient for them to be accorded symbolic power.

When I say that the substance was lacking, I am thinking particularly of the claim, implicit in the accounts offered by some mediators, that a perfunctory act of reparation is sufficient to generate forgiveness and reconciliation. This is counter-intuitive, as well as being at odds with the research evidence. Howard Zehr may well be right when he argues that victims need an experience of forgiveness (Zehr 1990), but, as he himself acknowledges, forgiveness does not come easily. It is not possible to forgive just because someone says 'sorry' – there has to be more of a relationship than that. As Thatcher likewise observes, remorse can only be manifested in the *totality* of changed behaviour, one part of which may be the verbal expression of regret . . . but 'no-one can expect verbal expressions of regret to be credible . . . unless they are accompanied by longer-term, non-verbal, tangible expressions of regret' (Thatcher 1991).

Whilst it is apparent that apology following serious injury may be interpreted differently in different cultures (Wagatsuma and Rosett 1986), any purported reparative action will be judged according to the weight of meaning which it carries within its own social context.

UK reparation schemes (and, it has to be said, some UK commentators) do not appear to recognise this. As a result, 'we are asked to accept . . . a flight of fantasy cloaked in a false aura of piety and saintliness' (Bayfield 1989). It may be desirable that victims forgive those who have injured them, but forgiveness has to be earned. As Bayfield goes on to explain:

> This is not a licence to harbour grudges and allow ill-will to fester, but a recognition of emotions whose acceptance is part of psychic health. Life demands that we move on, but moving on does not *ipso facto* imply we must go round exuding love and bonhomie for everyone who has harmed us, regardless of whether, given the chance, they would knowingly do it to us again. With characteristic realism, Jesus, *in extremis*, asked God to do the forgiving of people who knew not what they did.
>
> (Bayfield 1989)

These observations are borne out by research, although they might appear to be contradicted by the tone of the Marshall and Merry compilation. But Young's work at Coventry and Garton's at Leeds revealed, just as one might have expected, that although few victims saw value in imprisonment, 'most want(ed) some "upheaval" in the life of the criminal to compensate for the disruption to their (own) lives' (Garton 1986).

What this amounts to, in simple terms, is that victims want justice. Forgiveness may be possible, but only where justice is done. This is understood by that most persuasive advocate of restorative justice, Howard Zehr (1990). It is also a theme that imbues the writing of Stanley Cohen. Cohen describes how the various liberal, rehabilitative and reforming ideas can undermine what is due to the victim . . .

> Not rehabilitation, but justice has to be 're-affirmed', as an honourable moral value in itself and not merely something which the law mechanically requires . . . No organised system of justice can be constructed from the point of view of individual need and welfare.
>
> (Cohen 1985, p. 250)

It is especially regrettable that the practice of reparation schemes should be so vulnerable to these strictures. This is because reparation implies giving equal consideration to victim and offender, thereby satisfying our innate sense of rightness (Cohen 1985, p. 250). But if victims are merely to be used for the purpose of mitigation they will suffer further offence at the machinations of a system which retains its exclusive focus upon the offender. This does not mean that victims will be denied all consideration, but that they will continue to be pigeon-holed under that most revealing designation of inferior circumstance – 'victimology'. Any research to do with victims tends to be given this label. A study of assault victims, say, is unlikely to be seen as a way of exploring important issues concerning definitions of criminal behaviour or the delivery of criminal justice in our courts. Victimology pays scant regard to victims' greatest need, which is to be treated justly, and focuses instead upon an array of subsidiary needs – for support, courteous treatment, information, and so on. When Shapland contemplates a more victim-centred justice system, she does not envisage that the practice of courts might be fundamentally re-cast: 'The changes in the criminal justice system necessary to approximate more closely to the present expectations of victims are not major or structural ones' (Shapland 1984).

So victims are left with Criminal Injuries Compensation, the slim possibility of court-ordered compensation, and Victim Support. There are no vested interests calling for *more* than this; and to attempt to deliver more would run the risk of alienating those much more powerful forces whose life's work it is to judge, punish, and treat offenders. Reparation has now had its day as far as the Home Office is concerned. When, in 1988, this was put to the former head of the Research and Planning Unit, at the annual meeting of researchers and criminologists convened by the Home Office, she responded to the effect that 'we've heard enough about victims'. This was an interesting commentary upon the image of reparation held within that Unit. First, it confirmed the low priority accorded to the victim interest; but secondly, and more important, it revealed the short-comings of official imagination which could not conceive that research on victims might tell us something about the operation of the justice system as a whole.

Chapter 9

Victim–offender mediation in Germany

Heinz Messmer [1]

The first programmes of victim–offender mediation in the Federal Republic of Germany were set up in the mid 1980s, principally in the field of juvenile justice. There were several reasons for this. The German Juvenile Justice Act is based on the principle that educational goals should have priority over punishment. This reflects the view that juvenile offenders should not be regarded as fully responsible for their norm-violating behaviour, with no allowance made for their social circumstances. Nonetheless in practical terms the ascendancy of educational principles within juvenile justice remains precarious since there is no clear explanation of what is meant by education, nor of what this is intended to achieve. For example, punishment is often seen as a means of securing educational goals, suggesting that there is a blurring of boundaries. This vacillation between 'education' and 'punishment' reflects the fact that German juvenile justice has long been an area of experimentation in criminal justice policy. Victim–offender mediation is the latest of these experiments.

FIRST MODEL PROGRAMMES IN THE FEDERAL REPUBLIC OF GERMANY

Criticisms of punishment on the one hand and of educational initiatives on the other, together with increasing concern for the plight of crime victims, made German authorities receptive to the idea of restorative justice when reports were fed back from the USA and Canada in the early 1980s. The first programmes in the Federal Republic of Germany were set up in 1985: the 'Handshake' programme at Reutlingen; the 'Scales' programme at Cologne; victim–offender mediation in the juvenile court at Braunschweig (later extended to Munich and Landshut); and victim–offender mediation as part of a diversion programme at Bielefeld. The 'Handshake' and 'Scales' programmes are privately run, whilst the other experiments are run by established institutions serving the juvenile court.

The 'Handshake' programme dealt with 204 offenders in its experimental phase (June 1985 to December 1987). Most cases (57 per cent) involved more than one offence. The most common offence categories were theft, assault, and damage to property in the intermediate category (up to 500 German marks, or 170 pounds sterling, although 17 per cent of cases involved larger sums). Most of the offenders admitted to these programmes already had a criminal record. Seventy-two per cent of cases involved individual victims; institutions were victimised in 23 per cent; and the remaining cases were a mixture of the two (Kuhn et al, 1989, pp. 148ff).

At Cologne, the experimental phase (February 1986 to December 1988) covered 246 cases, involving 354 offenders and 363 victims. The main offence categories were assault, damage to property, fraud, and deception, with a tendency to include higher levels of loss or damage than at Reutlingen. Nearly half the offenders already had a criminal record. Seventy-five per cent of cases involved individual victims (Schreckling 1990, pp. 35ff).

A preliminary survey of mediation practice at Braunschweig (June 1986 to July 1987) indicated that, of 218 possible cases, 56 were referred by the juvenile court for victim–offender mediation. The majority of these concerned assault. There were a further 43 cases in which the court did not instigate mediation because restitution had been made beforehand, usually in cases of theft. Nearly twice as many offenders ($n = 29$) as victims ($n = 15$) declined to participate in mediation (Schmitz 1988, pp. 126ff).

The situation in the early days of the diversion programme at Bielefeld (January 1987 to May 1988) was comparable: although one-third of all 'diversion' cases appeared suitable for restitution ($n = 65$ offenders), a face to face meeting with a successful outcome occurred in less than 10 per cent. The difficulties at Bielefeld were the same as those at Braunschweig, apart from the latter's particularly high rejection rate amongst adolescent offenders. Between eighteen and forty cases were referred for victim–offender mediation each year. These mainly involved individual rather than corporate victims and the main offence category was assault, followed by theft and damage to property. In most cases an attempt was made to bring victim and offender face to face, but where there was a compensation claim (and the victim did not wish for anything else) agreement on this issue was considered sufficient.

Despite the above differences, it would seem that the casework in these experimental programmes is very similar. It is intended that the victim should be an individual, although corporate representatives are accepted; the facts of the crime should be agreed and the accused adolescent should have admitted guilt; petty offences, which are generally abandoned in current legal practice, should not be the object of mediation; on the other hand, the damage caused (particularly in respect of property) should not exceed the accused adolescent's restitutive capabilities; the participation of victim and offender is voluntary, at least formally speaking; victim and offender should resolve the issues at stake as directly and autonomously as possible; the discussion is intended to strengthen the young offender's sense of responsibility for the behaviour in question and for its consequences; the victim should explain the material and psychological consequences of the offence and use this as a basis to justify the claim for restitution; a figure for restitution cannot be imposed – it requires the approval of both parties; and restitution should replace punishment measures. With regard to case characteristics, only the clause excluding petty offences is problematic. This is because it is difficult to determine which cases would, in any event, be discontinued. This difficulty always arises when mediation is undertaken with a view to achieving diversion.

Referral to the 'Handshake' programme is the responsibility of the juvenile court service and takes place either after the charge has been put (but before the main court hearing) or before a charge has been preferred (Kuhn et al, 1989, p. 160). The Bielefeld programme secures its cases from the public prosecutor's office. The research revealed that Braunschweig performed two-thirds of its mediations before the court hearing and one-third afterwards (Schmitz 1988, p. 132). In contrast, the 'Scales' programme operated mainly within the framework of criminal prosecution, with 70 per cent of cases being referred by a judge. The Cologne programme was conducted mainly within the framework of court proceedings (approximately 60 per cent), or following the charge but prior to any hearing (Schreckling 1990, 41f; 107f).

All programmes declined to accept certain cases because of their petty character. There was little if any indication that minor matters, normally subject to diversion, were being drawn into the mediation net. For example, offenders in the 'Scales' programme at Cologne tended to have engaged in more serious crimes than had a control group of arrests (Schreckling 1990, 46f). Furthermore, amongst offences involving damage to property, victims referred to mediation secured an average restitution of 200 DM compared with 7 DM in the control group. In assault cases, victims referred to the 'Scales' programme secured an average 365 DM damages (31 DM in the control group) and 131 DM compensation (3 DM in the control group).

An important criterion of the success of the mediation programmes is their acceptance by the courts – in other words, an acceptance that mediation should secure diversion. In the 'Scales' programme at Cologne 72 per cent of mediation cases had the charges dropped. Of the remaining cases, in 61 per cent the only verdict was to confirm restitution, whilst in 39 per cent this was supplemented by further sanctions, mostly a caution, community work, or suspended detention. These court penalties were either a consequence of unsuccessful restitution, or of further offences, or they were imposed completely independently as an additional sanction (Schreckling 1990, pp. 109ff). In the 'Handshake' programme at Reutlingen restitution was the sole response in all but 7 per cent of cases (Kuhn et al, 1989, p. 193).

Whilst available data provide encouraging signs concerning the relationship between informal and formal justice, they also point to the complexity of this issue. As long as the relationship between criminal law and reparation models is not clearly structured, there remains a risk that mediation procedures will lead to net-widening. This is particularly true when individual model programmes (plus their attendant research) lose their exceptional status and become a scarcely controllable routine affair. This will be discussed later.

The available data on the success rates in mediation are promising. The proportion of successfully concluded mediations was 70 per cent in Munich and 57 per cent in Landshut. In the majority of cases a reparation agreement was based on a conversation between victim and offender, although in Munich reparation agreements were often mediated without any direct contact between the parties. The reparation agreed usually involved payment of compensation plus damages and symbolic gestures (Hartmann 1989). Research on the 'Handshake' programme distinguished between individual and corporate victims. The success rate with individuals was 78 per cent, with only 5 per cent of these cases not being dropped by the court. Amongst corporate victims the success rate was 92 per cent, of which

6 per cent were nevertheless processed formally. There was a direct contact between victim and offender in 59 per cent of cases involving an individual victim, but in only 21 per cent of cases involving a corporate victim. The usual forms of reparation were payment of compensation, followed by community work and the payment of damages (Kuhn et al, 1989, pp. 198ff). The 'Scales' programme at Cologne was deemed successful in over 70 per cent of cases, although only about a quarter of these involved direct contact between victim and offender. The dominant form of reparation was financial compensation (83 per cent), followed by apologies (29 per cent) and visits to the victim (17 per cent) (Schreckling 1990, pp. 78ff).

The first models of victim–offender mediation have now proved their worth in terms of their impact on legal practice. They are now accepted as a significant extension of the range of available responses. The privately run programmes at Cologne and Reutlingen have been consolidated, with some increases in personnel. The Bielefeld programme is striving within the framework of its diversion practice to increase the number of mediations. At Braunschweig efforts are currently directed towards implementing victim–offender mediation in adult as well as juvenile cases. It is estimated that one in three or one in four juvenile offences giving rise to a criminal charge may be suitable for victim–offender mediation. However, the referral rate in all programmes over the period of assessment was much lower (between 2 per cent and 8 per cent). Additional referrals, in terms both of crude numbers and broadened case characteristics, would seem to be both possible and desirable.

FUTURE PROSPECTS

'For juvenile offences in the Federal Republic of Germany . . . victim–offender mediation is at a threshold between isolated application in model programmes and its adoption into everyday law' (Schreckling 1990, p. 136). Even during the test phase of the above experiments, plans were being made to set up other mediation programmes aimed at both juveniles and adults. New programmes are being promoted at a national, regional, and community level. So one can say that after a relatively short trial period, victim–offender mediation has become an important element amongst the non-custodial measures currently available in juvenile justice. The discussion no longer concerns whether or not victim–offender mediation is appropriate and desirable; the main issues now concern its practical implementation. A recent amendment to the Juvenile Justice Act gave further encouragement to mediation by incorporating it into the diversion provisions of s.45 and s.47, thereby encouraging public prosecutors and judges to drop formal proceedings following the payment of damages. Mediation had also been incorporated into s.10 of the German Juvenile Justice Act, supplementing the range of non-custodial measures listed there.

Integration of victim–offender mediation into legal process nonetheless remains problematic. This is, first, because it is not easy to determine the priority which it should have; second, because s.10 of the German Juvenile Justice Act allows penalties to be combined, so there is a threat of multiple sanctioning; and third, because the widespread implementation of mediation would be very difficult to monitor and control. In addition, the mediation task calls for a high level of skill: this is incompatible with an uncontrolled, rapid growth in the number of schemes and personnel (Schreckling 1990, p. 137). In 1990 the German Probation Service conducted a survey of victim–offender mediation schemes in the Federal Republic. Approximately two thousand questionnaires were administered to legal and juvenile authorities and to various victim and offender assistance programmes. There were 1,252 replies, with 412 institutions (33 per cent of the sample) reporting that they were either directly or indirectly involved in the practice of victim–offender mediation, whilst a further 224 (18 per cent) were engaged in setting up or planning such a scheme. The majority of those addressing this task were youth authorities (69 per cent) and non-profit welfare organisations aiming to assist offenders and juveniles (21 per cent). Most of these organisations reported that victim–offender mediation was not their main field of work, but was rather seen as a subsidiary activity. Staff were seldom appointed specifically to engage in this task. Only eleven organisations reported that they dealt with between fifty and a hundred cases per annum, whilst only two dealt with more than a hundred.

Whilst this survey demonstrates the degree to which victim–offender mediation is now established, it also reveals serious difficulties. As long as mediation remains a marginal activity, as long as practitioners do not specialise in it, and as long as caseloads remain modest, then a further expansion of victim–offender mediation programmes carries considerable risk. One aspect of this has already been mentioned, namely, that measures of social control will be applied to cases that would otherwise have been dropped. Secondly, it is also conceivable that unsuccessful attempts at mediation will lead to harsher court penalties than if mediation had not been attempted. Thirdly, it is unclear whether the practice of mediation prior to a court decision violates the principle of assumed innocence. Fourthly, there are fears that victim–offender mediation might constitute a form of second-class justice in which the parties have inadequate legal protection, in which case these programmes might become a repository for troublesome disputes which are unwanted by the court. Fifthly, the fact that mediation is, for the most part, undertaken by agencies which have an offender orientation brings their neutrality into question: linking victim–offender mediation to the goals of diversion or decarceration involves a risk that the process will be biased in favour of the offender. Finally, mediation between victim and offender is a complex process which makes considerable demands upon the practitioner. It calls for the development of a bilateral conflict-solving paradigm which in turn involves a complex interaction for which there are, at present, few guidelines.

To advance victim–offender mediation will call for the mastery of four essential tasks over the coming years: further development; satisfaction of demand; quality control; and professionalisation (Schreckling 1990, pp. 138ff). The necessary steps are being campaigned for in Germany at the present time. An analysis of the scope for victim–offender mediation has already been conducted, as mentioned above. It is also proposed to set up a national 'centre for victim–offender mediation' with the task of advising new programmes and supporting their development through programme evaluation or supervision. Finally, a training programme for mediators is being prepared. Supported by the German probation service and the Association for Juvenile Courts and Juvenile Court Services, this will involve courses and workshops over a two-year period.

The need for training is clearly evident from the case studies contained in this volume. These reveal a great many errors, affecting the quality of the entire procedure: a frequently disproportionately puffed up procedural effort in response to petty offences; failure to inform the parties about the process; artificial conflict frameworks; a minor role for victims; poorly selected locations for the victim–offender meeting; no scope for the respective parties to articulate their grievances or to act together in conflict-solving; and an imbalance of power between victim and offender. Victim–offender mediation need not *necessarily* display these shortcomings, but such failings are always possible where there is a rapidly extended and uncontrolled application of an unfamiliar process.

VICTIM–OFFENDER MEDIATION AS AN INTERACTIVE PROCESS

Injustice is a product of social definitions and depends on how persons perceive and judge situations. The response to injustice can take many different forms. In modern societies a large part of this response occurs within formal court proceedings in which conflicts are decided with the help of normative constructs. These formal decisions follow a binary scheme: it is only possible to be in the right or in the wrong. Details of the parties' social circumstances and relationships have to be excluded until a point is reached when the offending behaviour can be assessed in relation to binding legal norms, whereupon a decision can be made. 'Law' is thus maintained through a decision-making process which need not be in accord with the psychological and social experience of the parties.

If one aspires to a justice process which makes sense to the parties, there are obvious difficulties in achieving this within the court setting, especially in the field of juvenile justice. If the decision-maker is less interested in consensus than in securing unequivocal, binding outcomes imposed within a set timetable, decision-making rules will dominate the proceedings. In contrast to the way in which conflict is resolved in everyday life, court procedure is dominated by rigid limitations which function primarily as speech barriers. Studies of communication in court have noted this imbalance, with the parties being seen as mere providers of information. Judicial authority, the ceremonies of the court, a lack of procedural flexibility, and lay people's ignorance of legal procedure all serve to promote uncertainty and powerlessness. Victim and offender alike have notably limited negotiating power before the court (Grümer 1984). Furthermore, it is known that the interrogative techniques of lawyers severely restrict the opportunities for lay persons to present their point of view, undermining any semblance of competence and objectivity in their speech (Atkinson and Drew 1979, passim). Psychological and social dimensions of their experience tend to be excluded. While a lay person may consider these facets of his experience to be important, lawyers have their own criteria of relevance. From the parties' perspective, justice and procedural rules often appear to be in conflict. In contrast, the attraction of victim–offender mediation rests, above all, on re-appraising deviant behaviour in the light of the parties' experience of the conflict and their needs thereafter. Ideally, this begins with their decision to participate in mediation, continues with individual judgements of the facts in question, and concludes with their acceptance of a reparation measure.

In the course of research on the Bielefeld diversion practice, discussions between social workers and their (young offender) clients were observed. Fifty-eight of these discussions were audio-taped, of which twenty-four were either preparatory to or included an attempt at mediation. All conversations were subject to content analysis and we conducted computer-assisted analysis of communication structures. In addition, twelve of these victim–offender mediations were fully transcribed. These transcripts revealed that juvenile offenders made full use of the chance to express their point of view. The fact that adolescents can speak freely in the context of an informal procedure made it possible to penetrate the superficial presentation of their deviant behaviour. The reasons for their having acted as they did were often clearly articulated. They generally knew very well that they had done something that they should not have done, but they were also capable of reflecting on the underlying causes of their behaviour and of rationalising this.

In many ways, a comparison can be drawn with the 'techniques of neutralisation' elaborated by Sykes and Matza (1957). Sykes and Matza observe that acceptance of a norm does not necessarily exclude its violation. The main function of these techniques, therefore, is to fend off accusations of injustice and reduce feelings of guilt by maintaining a positive self-image. A study of our transcripts revealed that many difficulties on the path towards agreement between victim and offender arose from the young person's ability to use injustice-neutralising justifications as a means of evading responsibility. Especially in relation to conflicts which have an interactive element, such as fights, it became clear that adolescents fall back on recurring justification strategies in order to counter their insight into the injustice committed.

Typically, the accused adolescent avoided taking responsibility, completely or partially, by blaming other factors in the conflict environment – mostly the opposing party. We have called such defensive techniques 'justification constructs'. This should make it clear that each has specific principles of construction which need not be presented immediately in discussion but which emerge step by step as they are referred to by those applying them. We were able to detect four types of justification, each of which differs somewhat from the techniques of neutralisation identified by Sykes and Matza. The first justification construct is grounded in a *competing version of the conflict*. In interpersonal conflicts it tends to be the beginning (and thereby the cause) that cannot be determined precisely. The typical justification employed is that of a normative disappointment prior to the officially recognised trigger event. This normative transgression is attributed to the opposing party, thereby legitimising the offender's aggressive act. In this way the young offender's own behaviour can be normatively enhanced while the behaviour of the opposing party is downgraded.

A second justification construct involves *competing norm concepts* and refers to the accused party's expectations concerning the behaviour of others. In victim–offender mediation there may be a tension between the offender's norm orientation and more conventional behavioural guidelines. The transcripts reveal that the accused adolescents tend to attribute normative deviance to the victim, he having failed to behave in a way which is consistent with the offender's own values. The victim is accused, for example, of violating principles of reciprocation, or of being disloyal. So the conforming and deviant elements in the behaviour are inverted: judged by the standards of the accused adolescent, it is the victim who has failed to behave correctly.

A third justification construct is *competing evaluations of the consequences of the deviant behaviour*. This involves casting doubt upon the alleged consequences of the offence, suggesting perhaps that these have been exaggerated by the victim. For example, we found that young offenders often accused their victims of being greedy for compensation, thus presenting themselves as the *real* victims since they suffered as a result of this mercenary attitude.

The fourth justification construct, *negative characterisation*, is applied to the personality of the victim. Aspects of the victim's behaviour are criticised, we suggest, in order to distract attention from the young offender's own behaviour. For example, the victim may be accused of avarice in seeking restitution. Negative characterisations of this kind may be seen as an attempt to undermine the credibility of the victim. This is another form of inversion, seeking to overturn our conventional judgements of good and bad behaviour.

These justifications 'neutralise' the impact of the deviant behaviour by suggesting alternative stories and interpretations. They also offer a system of beliefs and behavioural guidelines which provide support for this inversion process. The justifications aim to bridge the gap between what happened and what should have happened, between actual behaviour and accepted behavioural norms. They are designed to fend off stigma and achieve at least limited acceptance of the young person's deviance.

Victim–offender mediation therefore calls for a careful consideration of the conflict from the perspective of all those involved. This is the only way to ensure that these neutralising justifications are detected and that an agreement on restitution is not merely a response to the surface phenomenon of deviant behaviour. Instead, it should be a decision for which both parties accept responsibility and which, therefore, both mean to honour. The more conflict is articulated in all its aspects and the more it can be tackled through negotiation, the more likely it is that differences in the way the conflict is perceived will ultimately be bridged. Frank exchange is helpful in defining boundaries between acceptable and unacceptable behaviour, these boundaries being relevant to the problem in hand rather than mere abstractions. Although in one sense this gives rise to a further problem in that juvenile delinquents attempt to *justify* their behaviour (thus making agreement on reparation more difficult), this articulation provides an opportunity for mediator and victim to delve behind justification constructs in order to offer competing assessments. These in turn contribute to the offender's understanding that he has indeed behaved wrongly.

Conversation analysis revealed that the accused adolescents were capable of learning about their justification behaviour. This is apparent if preparatory talks between social workers and young offenders are compared with later mediations in the presence of victims. The adolescents often used the discussion which took place prior to mediation in order to construct a favourable negotiating position based on one or more of the justifications outlined above. As soon as they were given an opportunity to say what they thought about their behaviour, their motives, and the consequences of their actions, they attempted some rationalisation in order to neutralise the injustice committed. However, the presentation of their case focused the attention of the mediator and victim upon basic inconsistencies. Only when the offender's explanations had been discussed openly could they be used as a basis for further exploration and challenge. The research material reveals that even before direct confrontation between victim and offender, numerous weaknesses and inconsistencies could be identified in the justifications advanced. These could then be dealt with by the social workers. Direct contact between victim and offender further undermined the neutralisation effort: victims were particularly effective in counteracting those justifications which referred to what actually happened (competing versions of the conflict), the ensuing damages (competing evaluations of the consequences), and negative characterisations.

This evaluation of the impact of mediation is very much simplified in order to present an ideal standard of procedural justice that, although discernible in victim–offender mediation programmes, is generally not yet achieved in practice. The success of such programmes is not guaranteed by their goals. Nonetheless, there is reasonable hope that victim–offender mediation will stimulate problem-solving practices which transcend legal labels and allow access to the underlying causes of offending behaviour. If causes are to be addressed and effective intervention devised, we need the co-operation of the parties. Their definitions of the conflict are essential elements in arriving at appropriate responses. Negotiation in this context is both an instrument of intervention and a vehicle for assessment which makes it possible to decide upon other measures.

CONCLUSION

At times when traditional social values are under threat, it may seem increasingly difficult to understand the motivation of adolescents at a critical phase in their maturation. Law cannot concern itself with this. Underlying causes are excluded. The legal system sets clear priorities: the application of law comes first; justice is secondary. But, more than ever, we need to seek agreement on values and standards of behaviour. Deviant behaviour is not only a problem for society; it also reflects social relationships – and, as such, it is a problem for young offenders themselves. Our response to deviant behaviour needs therefore to be based on an analysis of norm orientations. These cannot be *imposed* if it is our intention to stimulate normative social behaviour. Christie has compared the acquisition of a sense of justice with the acquisition of language: although a person comes into this world with a predisposition both to speak and to have a sense of justice, each of these can be developed only in relationship with others (Christie 1982). In other words, each has to be *learnt*. Controller and controlled alike need to recognise what is cause and what is effect in order to achieve a proper solution to problems.

Accordingly, the correct response to deviant behaviour is not the application of law alone, but *the practice of fairness*. An important framework for this is provided by procedures in which the voices of the parties are heard and their norms taken into account. Despite the shortcomings necessarily associated with attempts to offer alternatives to law, these alternatives do have the advantage of allowing greater scope for communication between controller and controlled. Informal procedures help the participants understand the various causal relationships, so they gain insight into the real world of juvenile delinquency. These informal measures need to be applied to the causes, rather than to the manifestations of wrong-doing. Perhaps, in that way, we shall come to recognise that punishment is ineffective in changing behaviour.

NOTE

1 Thanks to Jonathan Harrow at the University of Bielefeld for the original translation of this paper.

Chapter 10

Victim–offender mediation
A review of research in the United States

Mark S. Umbreit and Robert B. Coates [1]

The practice of giving victims an opportunity to confront their offender in the presence of a mediator is a relatively new criminal justice reform effort in the US. By allowing victims and offenders to get answers to questions, to express their feelings, and to negotiate mutually acceptable restitution agreements, the victim–offender mediation process aims to enhance the experience of fairness for both offenders and victims. Despite more than ten years of programme development in the United States and a network of nearly a hundred programmes, there exist only a handful of empirical studies which assess the mediation approach. The aim of this chapter is to review all the major empirical studies of victim–offender mediation in the US. Key findings from each study will be presented, major themes identified, and implications for further research will be outlined.

It was not until 1974 that the specific intervention which, in the US, is called 'victim–offender reconciliation' was first attempted in North America in a small experiment in Kitchener, Ontario, at the initiative of representatives of the Mennonite church and a local judge and probation officer. Contact between victims and offenders had previously occurred in a number of programmes, most notably the nationally recognised Minnesota Restitution Center in Minneapolis. Mediation had also been employed at a pre-trial diversion stage. However, the victim–offender reconciliation process represented a significant extension of these other efforts in that it applied structured mediation techniques in a systematic fashion with convicted offenders and their victims, usually following offences of burglary and theft.

For the most part, victims and offenders involved in the programme had no prior personal relationship. Rather than focusing upon restitution, this first victim–offender reconciliation programme

(VORP) emphasised the need to address the emotional and informational needs of both parties through face to face mediation, with restitution representing an important additional goal. The VORP model was not simply an offender rehabilitation programme. Nor was it directed solely towards assisting the victim. Rather, it was designed to address the needs of the parties in a manner which rendered the justice process meaningful to both, enabling them to resolve the conflict in a manner which they considered appropriate, without court imposition (Umbreit 1985; 1986). The early success of the programme in Kitchener quickly led to replication in other parts of Canada.

The first replication of the VORP model in the United States occurred in 1978 in the northern Indiana community of Elkhart, once again through the leadership of the Mennonite church, this time acting in concert with a local judge, probation staff, and a local community corrections organisation called PACT (Prisoner and Community Together). This project in Elkhart came to receive nationwide and international attention from the criminal justice community (Umbreit 1988).

PROGRAMME RESEARCH

A national survey of victim–offender mediation programmes was conducted by Hughes and Schneider (1989). Questionnaires were sent to 171 programmes which reported that they conducted victim-offender mediation in cases involving juvenile offenders. Seventy-nine programmes, all having a victim–offender component, responded to the survey. Most were administered by private non-profit-making organisations, although a minority were run by probation departments or other public agencies. In just over 50 per cent of the programmes mediation was conducted solely by programme staff, but nearly 40 per cent of programmes also used volunteers. Less than 10 per cent of the programmes in the survey relied solely upon volunteer mediators. The most frequently cited component of reparation agreements negotiated in a mediation session was monetary restitution. Other elements that were mentioned, although less often, were community service, community service combined with restitution, and behavioural requirements of the offender, such as school attendance or counselling.

The VORP projects set up in the wake of the Elkhart initiative all received their cases from the courts, usually following conviction. A trained mediator would first meet separately with victim and offender in order to listen to their stories, explain the programme, and encourage their participation. If both agreed to take part, the mediator would then arrange a meeting at which the victim could ask questions and express his/her concerns directly to the person who had caused the injury. At the same time the offender had an opportunity to display a more positive side to his character. There would be an opportunity to negotiate restitution and plan repayment (Zehr and Umbreit 1982).

CONSUMER RESEARCH

The most informative study of victim–offender mediation and reconciliation was conducted by Coates and Gehm (1989) who evaluated VORPs in four Indiana communities. The researchers found that, for both victim and offender, being responded to as a person was probably the greatest strength of the programme. While some victims had chosen to participate in order that they might recoup their losses, they left feeling that they had been treated fairly and with dignity. Other findings were that offenders appeared to take the mediation process seriously and seemed to have a better sense that their action had hurt someone and required a response; victims placed considerable value on the opportunity for increased participation; a high proportion of restitution schedules were met in full by offenders; both victims and offenders viewed the programme as a legitimate form of punishment; and there was evidence to suggest that VORP, in conjunction with some short local jail time, was used as an alternative to more lengthy state incarceration in selected cases.

Eighty-three per cent of offenders and 59 per cent of victims expressed themselves satisfied with the VORP experience, with a further 30 per cent of victims being somewhat satisfied. Dissatisfaction was expressed by 11 per cent of victims, much of this having to do with the fact that they had not secured full restitution. If they had the opportunity again, 97 per cent of victims would choose to participate in VORP, and 97 per cent would likewise recommend VORP to other crime victims.

Victims identified the following as the most satisfying aspects of the process:

1. the opportunity to meet the offender in order to obtain a better understanding of the crime and of the offender's situation;

2. the opportunity to secure restitution;
3. the offender's expression of remorse;
4. the care and concern of the mediator.

The researchers note that 'it is interesting that more victims commented on meeting with the offender than on restitution, given that the number one reason for most victims choosing to participate in the first place was financial restitution'. Aspects of the process that victims found least satisfying were:

1. lack of adequate follow-up and leverage on the offender to fulfil the agreed contract;
2. the delay between offences and resolution through the VORP process;
3. the amount of time required to participate in VORP.

From the offender's perspective, the most satisfying elements were:

1. meeting the victim and discovering that the victim was willing to listen to them;
2. staying out of jail and in some instances escaping a criminal record;
3. the opportunity to work out a realistic schedule for restitution and 'make things right'.

The researchers found that an offender would often regard meeting the victim as both the most satisfying and yet the least satisfying aspect of the experience. They suggest that this reflects the tension between, on the one hand, the stress experienced in preparing for the meeting, and, on the other, relief at having taken steps 'to make things right'.

For victims and offenders who participated in a face to face meeting there was a high probability that restitution contracts would be agreed (98 per cent) and completed (82 per cent of financial and 90 per cent of service agreements). Seventy-nine per cent of victims and 78 per cent of offenders believed that justice had been done in their case. Coates and Gehm (1989) concluded that 'the VORP process encourages personal accountability on the part of the offender while breaking down stereotypes of both offenders and victims. To the extent that it is desirable to personalize crime and justice, the VORP approach has much to offer'.

Gehm has also studied factors affecting victim willingness to participate in mediation (Gehm 1990). He analysed data from six victim–offender reconciliation programmes in Indiana, Minnesota, Oregon and Wisconsin. Three factors emerged as significantly affecting the victim's decision to participate in mediation. Victims were more likely to accept a face to face meeting if the offender was white; if the crime that had been committed was a misdemeanour (that is to say, relatively minor); and if the 'victim' was an institution such as a school or church, rather than someone victimised in their own person. Gehm notes, however, that these findings must be regarded with caution since there were relatively few minority victims in his sample.

Victims' experience of fairness within the mediation process has been examined by Umbreit (1989; 1990). The research comprised fifty interviews with burglary victims in Hennepin County, Minnesota, all of whom were referred, in 1986/7, to a VORP run by the Minnesota Citizens Council on Crime and Justice. Thirty-one of these victims (62 per cent) had participated in a mediation session with the offender. The remainder chose not to enter the mediation process. In each of these fifty cases the offender was a juvenile. VORP gave these burglary victims an opportunity to confront their offender in the presence of a trained mediator so that they could talk about the offence, express their concerns, and negotiate a mutually acceptable restitution agreement. The interviews revealed that ideas about 'fairness', as expressed by these burglary victims, principally reflected a restorative rather than retributive paradigm. In fact there were three main concerns: punishment of the offender; compensation of the victim; and rehabilitation of the offender. These concerns were expressed by 62 per cent of victims who participated in mediation and 38 per cent of those who did not. The response which was expressed most frequently and intensely concerned the offender's need for rehabilitation services such as counselling, family therapy or educational assistance. This concern was expressed by all those victims who participated in mediation and by 90 per cent of those who did not. Compensation for losses was the second most frequently expressed concern. The need to punish the offender through some form of incarceration was the point of view *least* frequently expressed.

A major factor determining these burglary victims' satisfaction with the response to their victimisation was the extent to which they were enabled to participate in the justice process. This included both passive forms of participation (information provided by letter) and active forms (court appearance and/or mediation). Ninety-seven per cent of victims considered that they had been treated fairly in the mediation session; 93 per cent held that the restitution agreement was fair; and 86 per cent said that they had found it helpful to meet the offender in order to discuss the offence and negotiate restitution. Victims who had opted to participate in mediation were twice as likely as non-participants to consider that they had been fairly treated within the justice process as a whole (80 per cent as against 38 per cent). This certainly suggests that the mediation process, with its opportunities for empowerment, contributes to crime victims' experience of fairness.

The author subsequently conducted post-mediation interviews with a further sample of fifty-one victims and sixty-six juvenile offenders drawn from the Center for Victim Offender Mediation in Minneapolis (Umbreit 1991). Of the 379 cases referred to CVOM in 1989, 50 per cent resulted in face to face mediation, 9 per cent in indirect mediation, and 41 per cent were referred back to the court. The main reasons why mediation did not take place were that the victim was unwilling (35 per cent); offender was unwilling (24 per cent); or the conflict was resolved by the parties prior to referral (17 per cent).

These interviews again revealed a high level of satisfaction with the mediation process on the part of both victims and offenders. Victims who met 'their' offender indicated that being able to talk about what happened and express their concerns was more important than receiving compensation for their losses. While 75 per cent of victims stated that receiving restitution was important, 90 per cent indicated that other, non-monetary benefits were of greater significance. As with the previous study, some 80 per cent of victims expressed concern about the offender's need for counselling and/or other rehabilitative services.

When crime victims were asked what they liked most about mediation, three themes emerged. First, telling the offender how the crime had affected them emotionally and/or financially was important. 'It was a chance to tell the offender the hardship it put on us as a family.' 'It was important to just let him know what he put me through, that it was more than one person he victimized.' A second theme concerned the importance of directly confronting the offender. 'I liked that the kid had to look me in the eyes.' 'I guess being able to meet him face to face and realize that he was just a kid who made a mistake was what I liked the most.' The third theme was victims' concern to help the person who had victimised them. 'I wanted most of all to help the boy.' 'The programme helps the offender to make restitution and I feel better knowing [the offender] will get help.' 'Confronting their victims could straighten the kids out.'

Ninety per cent of victims were happy with their experience of the programmes and nearly all felt that the restitution agreement was fair to both sides. Most victims (55 per cent) emerged with a positive attitude towards 'their' offender. Ninety-four per cent said they had no fear of further victimisation by that person. The only aspects of the mediation programme which victims said they disliked were the anxiety which they experienced beforehand . . . 'the unknown of the meeting, not knowing what they'd be like', and the initial tension in the mediation session, as indicated by statements such as 'I felt nervous'; 'it was a very tense situation'.

The young offenders who engaged in the mediation process were also, broadly speaking, satisfied with the experience. Telling the victim what happened, working out an acceptable restitution plan, making restitution, apologising – all these were regarded, by the great majority of offenders, as valuable components of the process. Ninety-five per cent of the offenders in this study actually offered an apology to their victim. Overall, offenders indicated a slightly lower level of satisfaction with the mediation experience than did their victims. For example, almost all victims indicated that the restitution agreement was fair to both parties, whereas just 88 per cent of offenders considered that the agreement was fair to them. The picture was still a positive one, however, with over 90 per cent of these young offenders believing that it was helpful to have met their victim. The value of getting to know the victim and discovering that he/she was a pleasant person who understood them were two of the most common themes. There was also reference to the quality of communication. 'I liked the honesty.' 'It was good to be able to actually say how you felt about it.' 'I liked that we could talk and get things out in the open.' Being able to apologise, having the chance to tell the victim what happened, and working out a restitution plan were other important although less frequently expressed themes.

As with the victims whom we interviewed, the aspect of the experience most disliked by these young offenders was the anxiety which they experienced prior to and during the meeting. 'It was hard meeting him face to face.' 'It was kind of scary and nerve-racking.' 'Before I met him it was scary.' 'I didn't like the beginning of the meeting because you are so afraid.' 'I felt kind of stupid and guilty because he was real sad . . . but it felt better after I had a chance to apologise.'

Reference should also be made to an earlier study which saw one of the few attempts to conduct a controlled experiment aimed at measuring the impact of mediation. This research took a sample of cases referred by the criminal courts in New York (Davis 1980). It studied a unique project in New York City which dealt primarily with cases arising from felony arrests, usually assault or burglary. This fact set the Brooklyn Dispute Resolution Center apart from the other mediation and conflict resolution programmes being established throughout the country, nearly all of which would not even consider felony arrests. The Brooklyn experiment also differed from other programmes offering victim–offender mediation in that (a) all offenders referred to it were diverted from prosecution; and (b) the parties had an ongoing relationship. Sponsored jointly by the Institute for Mediation and Conflict Resolution in New York City and the Victim/Witness Assistance Project of the VERA Institute of Justice, the Brooklyn Dispute Resolution Center mediated or arbitrated disputes between persons who knew each other, these disputes having erupted into criminal offences for which arrests were made. The mediation process was offered to the parties as an alternative to the conventional process of prosecution in Brooklyn Criminal Court.

An evaluation of this project by Davis (1980) focused upon a comparison of mediation and prosecution as they affected the parties' satisfaction with the process by which their cases were resolved. The extent to which hostilities recurred was also examined. Arrests which were screened as appropriate for mediation were randomly assigned into either a control or an experimental group. In comparing the experimental and control groups, Davis found that 'it was apparent that complainants whose cases were referred to mediation felt they had greater opportunity to participate in the resolution of the dispute, felt that the presiding official had been fairer, and felt that the outcome was more fair and more satisfactory to them'. Similar responses were given by defendants. However, the research found no indication that further conflict between the participants was less frequent among cases referred to mediation than among those subject to formal court intervention.

This brings us to the question of recidivism rates following mediation, a topic which has been very little studied in the US. Apart from the Davis research there appear to be only two investigations which bear on this subject. Guedalia (1979) found that offender contact with their victims correlated with a reduction in recidivism among juvenile offenders in Tulsa County, Oklahoma. This was despite the fact that 'victim contact' was limited to a meeting or to the delivery of a letter of apology. There was no victim–offender mediation as such. Schneider (1986) found that mediation was associated with a significant reduction in recidivism rates (from 63 per cent to 53 per cent) among juvenile offenders in Washington, D.C. This was a controlled study of two groups of offenders, one group having participated in a restitution programme based on mediation while the other had been assigned to the standard form of probation supervision. These were all serious felony offenders, with over 60 per cent being repeat offenders. A complicating factor, however, was that those offenders who were referred to mediation but chose not to participate (40 per cent of that group) also had a lower recidivism rate than those offenders randomly assigned to probation. Viewed most positively, this finding might be taken to suggest that even to allow juvenile offenders a say in the way their case is handled has some positive impact upon their future behaviour.

CONCLUDING REMARKS

The relatively few empirical studies examining victim–offender mediation in the US paint a favourable picture with regard to such matters as client satisfaction with the process, perceptions of fairness, and (in so far as it has been studied) impact upon recidivism. These studies do, however, have significant limitations. For example, virtually all the client satisfaction data reported by Coates and Gehm (1989) and Umbreit (1988; 1989; 1990) is presented without examining its relationship to a control group of victims and offenders who did not participate in the mediation process. While it is helpful to know that there is this degree of satisfaction among victims and offenders who participate in mediation, further controlled studies might prove even more enlightening. Furthermore, while the Guedalia and Schneider studies suggest that contact between victim and offender may reduce recidivism, neither study demonstrates the impact of the mediation process specifically. The Guedalia study involved only very limited contact between victim and offender, while in the Schneider study the data suggest that the fact that offenders were granted a choice may have had as much impact as the mediation process itself.

In future research it will be important to conduct more sophisticated studies of client satisfaction and perceptions of fairness, controlling for key variables such as age, race, sex, category of offence, and prior involvement with the courts. The issue of restitution completion by offenders who experience mediation, as compared with similar offenders ordered to pay restitution by a court, also needs to be examined. Finally, there need to be further studies of recidivism amongst offenders who participate in mediation. Such an analysis should include multiple measures of recidivism in order to determine the frequency, intensity, and severity of any further criminal behaviour.

NOTE

1 Part of the data reported in this chapter was made possible by a grant from the State Justice Institute in the US. Points of view expressed within this chapter are those of the authors and do not necessarily represent the official position of the State Justice Institute.

Chapter 11

Conclusion

It is difficult to conceive of a significantly increased reparative element within criminal justice, let alone the adoption of a 'new paradigm' (Zehr 1990), because we are so conditioned to the justice system as it is. As Priestley and McGuire have observed (1985, p. 214), common sense assessments of criminal justice cannot be relied upon because present practice is hidden beneath 'the accretion of several centuries of custom and usage, and of an elaborate theory that places the law in the realm of metaphysics, above mere reason and certainly above politics'. This makes life difficult for reformers, not least because they are unsure how ambitious they should be. The most radical theorists inevitably offer few signposts to a new practice, whilst reform initiatives can appear plodding, marginal and mundane.

And yet the failure of our procedures and punishments to meet their declared objectives has been almost universally acknowledged (Campbell 1984). To many of the standard criticisms, such as the difficulty in constructing a coherent philosophical defence of retribution and the failure of deterrence and rehabilitation, Nils Christie has added several more imaginative ones (Christie 1977, 1982, 1986). He points to the 'theft' of many conflicts (which he suggests are an essential social lubricant) by professional practitioners – lawyers and social workers. This is a loss to victims and offenders alike since they are denied an opportunity to define the nature of their own quarrel or to resolve it in ways that make sense to them. The almost total exclusion of the victim from the court process means that justice is inevitably cast in terms of retribution; there can be no discussion of what might be done 'to undo the deed' (see also Shapland et al, 1985, p. 188).

Victims' lack of involvement in the justice process – and the fact that society's interest is represented exclusively by professionals – means that offenders are more than ever reviled and feared. The powerful symbolism of the court ensures that they are seen as entirely different from the rest of us. This sense of psychological and social distance fuels a demand for more punitive action, while offenders who are on the receiving end of such painful treatment feel only resentment (Priestley 1977). This 'treatment' is also contemptuous in that it reflects an assumption that serious offenders have nothing to offer but their liberty . . . 'We let the poor pay with the only commodity that is close to being equally distributed in society: time. Time is taken away to create pain' (Christie 1982).

Two of Christie's themes are central to the case for a reparative component within criminal justice. The first concerns the lack of drama in our courts and hence the failure of Western-style justice to achieve psychological relevance; and the second has to do with the relationship between utilitarianism and excessive pain delivery. I shall summarise each in turn.

Most criminal cases stir hardly any emotion in the courtroom (Balint 1951). The professional participants are not emotionally engaged and there is generally no audience. The result is an unconvincing theatrical performance, bordering on hypocrisy. It is inevitable in these circumstances that offenders will feel persecuted rather than remorseful. Professional domination of the proceedings and the deliberate refusal to countenance ambiguity or lay accounts mean that there is, as Balint puts it, no effective psychotherapy – for the offender, for the victim (who is of course not present), or for the rest of us (likewise not present since we anticipate, all too accurately, that we would be both uncomprehending and uninvolved). The emotional flatness engendered by professional language and legal classification make punishment easy, because apparently scientific, whilst leaving on one side difficult and dramatically interesting questions concerning accountability and possible repair.

Christie's second point concerns the harmful consequences of inflicting punishment with a view to achieving social control. He emphasises that punishment must be understood, without euphemism, as the deliberate infliction of pain (see also Cohen 1985, p. 253). But utilitarianism obscures this basic truth. Punishment which is delivered through representatives and is intended to serve a purpose extraneous to the parties (for example, to convey a message to other potential offenders) may be both arbitrary and excessive. Christie therefore argues for less 'objectification' of the process of punishment: punishment which is not designed to do anything other than make sense to the parties will lead to a reduction in the amount of pain imposed (Christie 1982 and 1986). The case for a purely expressive or absolute view of punishment is also adopted by Garland (1990, p. 291) who concludes that 'the institutions of punishment should be seen – and should see themselves – as institutions for the expression of social values, sensibility, and morality, rather than as instrumental means to a penological end'.

If we view punishment in this light it becomes possible to conceive of a substantial reparative element within what is otherwise a retributive system of justice (Watson et al, 1989). There is, in particular, a sophisticated philosophical defence of retribution which advocates of reparative justice might also employ. This is the moral education theory (Moberly 1968; Hampton 1984) which holds that punishment is a means of teaching a wrong-doer that an action is morally wrong. (The lesson is public, and so is also directed at the rest of society.) The theory assumes that there is an identifiable right and wrong; and that human beings are autonomous. This view of punishment acknowledges the wrong suffered by the victim: the punishment is a reflection of this since it is taken to 'represent' the victim's suffering. But because such punishment is intended to convey a moral message, it must not itself be cruel. It is only justified as an attempt to improve a wayward person. But the offender must accept this justification if the reformative potential is to be realised; failing that, any punishment will be dismissed as vindictive.

It is not difficult to discern the relevance of this theory to the various attempts at reparative justice which we have been studying. Direct contact between offender and victim, or services performed for the victim, may be an even more effective means of conveying this same moral message. These requirements are also less likely to threaten the offender's future since they do not have the expelling character of imprisonment (Walgrave 1991). Furthermore, moral education theory points up the mistake of seeking to *coerce* repentance – whether such coercion is attempted by courts, reparation schemes, or by some administrative authority such as the parole board. This is manipulation *of* the offender – and it in turn invites manipulation *by* the offender. No moral message is conveyed (except perhaps that duplicity is rewarded), so there is little prospect of reform.

Reference to administrative authority is important in this context because it should remind us of the increasing tendency for key decisions in the penal process to be taken by administrators, acting on their executive power, following an administrative rather than a judicial logic (Garland 1990, p. 188). This partly arises from resource problems and the accompanying need to control expenditure from the centre. As a result our justice apparatus has as much an administrative as a judicial character. One aspect of this is the commitment to diversion from the court process, a policy pursued most enthusiastically in relation to juveniles (Davis et al, 1989). Diversion is commonly regarded as providing an opportunity for reparative initiatives, but it might equally be viewed as *denying* such an opportunity in that it reflects an administrative ethic to which reparative considerations, even more than retributive ones, will be rendered subservient (Davis et al, 1988). A non-utilitarian conception of punishment might render obsolete the commitment to diversion whilst allowing greater scope for justice expressed in reparative terms.

Much the same point might be made in relation to the management of criminal cases by the legal profession and the courts. What courts aspire to, above all, is the efficient processing of an uncomfortably large volume of cases. The behaviour in question will already have had an offence label attached to it; the great majority of offenders plead guilty. Just as with diversion, plea-bargaining at the door of the court may be regarded as antithetical to the principles of reparative justice rather than as a vehicle for their achievement. That is not to say that every minor transgression should be accorded all the trappings of due process; but it is more disturbing to subvert reparative considerations to an administrative ethic than it is to subvert demands for retribution. This is because there is a liberal consensus that we deliver too much pain in any event, whereas the victim interest cannot be dismissed so lightly.

This brings me to an important paradox at the heart of the vision of reparative justice advanced by Nils Christie (see also Thatcher 1991), namely, that concern for offenders is as important as concern for victims and that we shall achieve a *less* punitive reaction to offenders if victims are granted a major role in the justice process. Advocates of diversion and, it has to be said, some practitioners within reparation schemes appear to be afraid of victims. Victim involvement, it is assumed, will lead to offenders being punished more severely. In fact, the opposite may be true. To give greater priority to the needs of victims may make it more difficult for us to sustain our present depersonalised stance towards offenders – and it is this psychological distance which enables us to punish severely. It is one of the weaknesses of the present system that victim compassion and decency, just as much as victim suffering, is excluded from the court process.

REPARATION WITHIN RETRIBUTIVISM

Profound hostility has been expressed to the notion that victim–offender mediation and reparation might have a bearing upon the justice meted out within our criminal courts (see, for example, Powell 1985). One can see why such considerations might appear unduly subjective and therefore anomalous (Campbell 1984), but they can equally be regarded as an attempt to place criminal acts in their proper context of social and personal relationships. This suggests a move away from a rigid categorisation of offences and a greater emphasis on *stories* (as recounted by both victim and offender). Justice would no longer be neat and tidy, but, as Campbell says, it might be more realistic and defensible. In that case, the relationship between reparation and punishment would be much clearer than under the practice of present-day reparation schemes in England and Wales. Far from being designed to divert or mitigate, reparation would *be* the punishment (in whole or in part). To this might be added retributive punishment, if deemed necessary, and reformative initiatives, if thought appropriate (Christie 1977). Implicit in this proposal is an understanding that reparation contains an element of punishment – that it generally has some *cost* to the offender, whether this be reflected in loss of face or in the giving of time or money.

It is precisely for this reason that retributivism as we experience it in the West already allows reparative considerations to enter in. Whilst the aim of arriving at a level of punishment which is proportionate to the seriousness of the offence lies at the heart of our justice system, courts are also willing to be impressed by other considerations – many of them contained within the apparently unified concept of reparation. For example, they are willing to be impressed by the restitutive element, the rehabilitative element, the reconciliation element, or the contrition element – whatever they choose to see as contained within a particular act of reparation. The essentially retributive nature of our justice process is revealed in the experience of some reparation schemes that courts seek evidence that the reparation process is difficult; that it hurts. But courts are also willing to be influenced by suggestions that the reparative act has brought about some change in the attitude of the offender; that the needs of the victim have to some extent been met; or that the offender shows remorse. To this extent, therefore, reparation schemes are pushing against an open door. This, needless to say, does not herald a new vision of criminal justice; indeed, the whole point is that it is *not* new. As Blagg has observed: 'The present system would surely manage to assimilate material restitution within an unreformed punishment paradigm' (Blagg 1986).

However, it is as well to remind ourselves that some forms of reparation *cannot* readily be incorporated within court-based criminal justice. This is because the harm done is never confined to a person's body or property; it also involves damage to a social and moral relationship (Watson et al, 1989). The offender's action implies lack of concern for, perhaps even denial of, the victim's right to security in his or her person or possessions. So reparation, if it is to be complete, must make some attempt to make amends for the victim's loss of the presumption of security. This can only be remedied by some effort to reassure the victim that his or her rights are now respected. This point is crucial for discussion of the relationship between reparation and a retributive criminal justice system. One component in reparation cannot be coerced. Trust that the appropriate moral standards are shared by the offender cannot be restored by a court order requiring the offender to share those standards. If the victim is to be reassured, he or she must believe that the attitude in question is freely expressed. This, then, is a component in reparation which can only be achieved by the parties themselves, perhaps with the aid of some agency which lacks a court's coercive power.

INFORMAL NEGOTIATION

It is equally important to consider *the means* by which a change of attitude may be brought about – and here Heinz Messmer's research offers important clues. Through his examination of an alternative form of conflict resolution Messmer points up the general inability of criminal courts to fulfil anything other than an expressive purpose. Courts impose rigid speech barriers; victim and offender alike have very little negotiating power; underlying causes are excluded; justifications are seldom advanced – and if they are advanced, cannot be explored. Legal decision-making cannot therefore take account of the parties' sense of justice. The *rules* for decision-making – that is to say, legal procedures – dominate the courtroom. These procedures are inflexible, inhibiting normal discourse . . . 'In court, conflicts are generally neither mediated nor solved, but decided on' (Messmer 1989). In these circumstances it is only to be expected that offenders remain preoccupied with their own fate. Their defence mechanisms ('techniques of neutralisation' as theorised by Sykes and Matza, or 'justifications' according to Messmer) are not challenged effectively.

Informal procedures, on the other hand, allow the parties to a conflict to voice their own concerns and express their own values. The response to deviant behaviour needs to be couched in terms of those values if there is to be any prospect of a change in attitude or behaviour. The application of law cannot of itself achieve this; justice also has to be *perceived*. It is Messmer's thesis that this 'practice of fairness' can only be achieved in an informal setting. The negotiations which he describes are arduous and time-consuming, but they nonetheless offer an attractive model, one in which '(j)ustice is not only applied, but also learned' (Messmer 1991).

Possible reservations concerning this form of negotiation centre upon the willingness of 'victims' and 'offenders' to engage in the process and, secondly, the availability of skilled mediators. Most every-day conflict is dealt with by absorption – by 'lumping it'. Mediation does not appear to be the preferred method of conflict-resolution in our culture. It is salutary to recall Auerbach's observation, made in the context of an attempt to introduce conciliation as an alternative to small claims courts in the USA: 'The appeal of conciliation (to lawyers) was evident. But there was a fatal flaw in its theory and practice: it was alien to its presumed beneficiaries' (Auerbach 1983, p. 100). I would not wish to suggest that the negotiations which Messmer describes are alien to those who participate in them, but at the moment at least it is not how we do things. This was likewise Merry's conclusion in relation to community dispute-resolution in the USA: 'American communities are not structured to assume the social control functions currently performed by the legal system in a way which would genuinely decentralise control of behaviour' (Merry 1989).

Other commentators, for example Stanley Cohen, regard the renewed interest in mediation as indicative of 'a profound sense of nostalgia' in which a (real or imagined) past community is seen as providing the ideal form of social control: 'The iconography is that of the small rural village in pre-industrial society, in contrast to the abstract, bureaucratic, impersonal city of the contemporary technological state' (Cohen 1985, p. 117). This criticism cannot fairly be applied to Messmer's accounts since these are free of any spurious evocation of 'community', but it has to be admitted that the mediation and reparation literature is full of such references. This is despite the fact that these initiatives are almost invariably run by state agencies. As Cohen sardonically observes: 'Most attempts to recreate community in fact constitute evidence of the *end* of community. The central impurity at the heart of the community control ideology lies in the role of the state' (1985, p. 123). Nowhere do these strictures apply with greater force than in relation to reparation schemes in England and Wales, most of which were controlled by the Home Office and managed by the probation service.

The charge that 'community' initiatives in fact represent an extension of state power is by now a familiar one and in a sense all too easy to make. The same might be said of the claim that informal processes come to replicate all the features (including the social control obligations) of the formal systems which they were intended to replace (Merry 1989). Almost any initiative within criminal justice has the potential to be oppressive, but if mediation and reparation schemes addressed the concerns of the parties, rather than simply reflecting the traditional preoccupations of the liberal wing of the social control business, then perhaps we should suspend our cynicism. It cannot be right to treat offenders as if they have no moral sense and yet, with our combination of retribution and welfare, that is what we tend to do. But we need to be careful in defining the circumstances in which mediation is to be attempted (Messmer's focus, after all, is relatively narrow in that he is primarily concerned with fights). I agree with Christie (1982) that the objective should always be to respond in ways that make sense to the parties – in other words, to try to create 'a familiar landscape'. Mediation and reparation schemes offer the prospect of achieving this in some instances, whereas retributivism (and, I should say, diversion) all too often fail to generate any sense of rightness.

REFLECTIONS UPON REPARATION INITIATIVES IN THE UK

The recent history of reparation in England and Wales is that of a hastily conceived, under-theorised 'initiative' which was then further hampered by a lack of effective co-ordination between the Home Office and the various experiments which it was sponsoring.

These schemes developed a practice and philosophy which had not been anticipated by their political masters and which, when it was understood by them, did not appeal. This failure of co-ordination and lack of interest in one another's purposes was revealed, all too starkly, in the response to the Home Office discussion document (1986). The Home Office was interested in the introduction of a low-level court penalty, either alongside or integral to probation, as a further alternative to imprisonment. Reparation schemes, on the other hand, were seeking to distance themselves from the formal justice process (FIRM 1986). The fact that the Director of FIRM at that time was on secondment from the Home Office Research and Planning Unit, where he had been responsible for co-ordinating research into reparation schemes, only added to the poignancy of this situation.

It was inevitable, in these circumstances, that government interest in reparation would shrivel and die. When it became evident that reparation schemes wanted to do their own thing, the Home Office withdrew. By 1986, Leon Brittan and David Mellor, the Home Office ministers principally identified with the reparation initiative, had moved on. The new Home Secretary, Douglas Hurd, announced that he would await the results of the experiment then being conducted before taking any further action (results whose publication was delayed until 1990). At the end of 1986, a senior civil servant told Paul Rock, then researching victim support schemes, that 'reparation is a dead duck' (Rock 1990, p. 401). This was an inglorious end to a policy initiative which revealed all the weaknesses of the self-confident approach to policy-making characteristic of British politicians and civil servants (Thomas 1986).

It is worth reviewing the most fundamental defects.

Marginalisation

Reparation schemes were marginalised by courts, by police, and by lawyers. This was reflected in the relationship of schemes to the court and, in particular, in the supplicatory position in which they were placed, or placed themselves. Reparation was extraneous to the main business of the court – something which might be allowed to become a factor in mitigation. It was largely restricted to minor offences, or to disposals in which it might add to the repertoire of means used to achieve other purposes. Its relationship to the court process was tenuous and in many cases appeared designed to be ritualised, perfunctory and 'symbolic' (although it is a tribute to the vigour with which some mediators pursued their goal of offender education and attitude change that the process did rise above this on occasions). Even in those comparatively few cases in which reparation was attempted, one could not say that private conceptions of the harm done, or of what was necessary to make it right, weighed very significantly alongside the state-imposed tariff. A gloomy view would be that the marginalisation of reparation was confirmed, and perhaps even reinforced, by the development of out of court schemes which were treated with varying degrees of condescension by most legal personnel.

Ambiguity

Reparation in England and Wales was marked by ambiguity of objective, ambiguity of process, and ambiguity in the relationship between reparation schemes and the court. There was a very uneasy accommodation between court-based retribution and semi-independent reparation. Many proponents of reparation were principally interested in diversion, or in the imposition of less severe punishments, but they feared that they would have difficulty in convincing police and magistrates of their case. So they invited offenders to jump through hoops which they believed to be consistent with the values of those key decision-makers. Because these performances were not scrutinised, because their perfunctory nature was not acknowledged, and because police and courts are themselves not convinced of the value of punishment in some instances, reparation schemes did indeed have some marginal impact upon prosecution and sentencing decisions. But this was at a considerable cost in that they were viewed by courts as merely contributing to the mitigation process. (This is hardly surprising given that victims were never present in court to give their account of whether or not a degree of reparation had in fact been achieved.) It also meant that reparation was marginalised even within the practice of the schemes themselves. In other words, the pursuit of voluntary (and not self-interested) reparation – which would have been the strength of any scheme which was truly independent of the court – was undermined by the strenuous efforts which *were* made to get courts to take account of whatever vestigial element of reparation had been performed.

Inversion

There has developed, in Britain and the USA, a curious distinction between restitution and compensation (the language is American, but the thinking is common to both countries). Restitution has come to be regarded as an offender-orientated measure (Hudson and Galaway 1977). It may involve payment to the victim, or services to a substitute 'victim', but 'while restitution as a theory clearly has the victim in mind, its primary interest has remained the offender' (McAnany 1978). In Britain and the USA, reparation schemes (or 'restitution programmes') select cases on the basis of offender merit and need, the victim's needs being secondary if not incidental. The term 'victim compensation', on the other hand, is confined, in the USA, to payments made to victims by the state. In Britain our use of the term is not restricted in this way, but we do have the distinction in practice. (In both countries, state compensation tends to be limited to crimes of violence, whereas offender restitution is usually imposed in response to crimes of property.) This view of restitution as being geared to the offender interest means that it is difficult to incorporate it within a retributive justice model. This would *not* be the case were we to ascribe to the terms 'reparation' and 'restitution' their literal meaning, as indicating some contribution to making good the harm done. But the dominant characteristic of reparation schemes is their desire to appease a punishing system. So information which might convey an unfavourable impression of the offender is glossed over, whilst considerable significance is attached to even the most perfunctory act of reparation. Many practitioners within reparation schemes are, it is true, attracted by the idea of making amends. But they (or their predecessors) have traditionally been preoccupied with diversion and mitigation. Those concerns have been allowed to take precedence. As a result, these same practitioners are only weakly committed, if at all, to the idea that victims have a *right* to reparation, or that offenders have an *obligation* to repair.

Limited relevance

It has been observed that the practice of mediation has an astructural bias in that it typically fails to address the broad social factors which give rise to conflict or impede its resolution (Mika 1991). This criticism is applied to mediation in the USA, but it is equally valid in relation to reparation schemes in England and Wales. This is because, in seeking to serve the court and to reflect the court's values, reparation schemes have adopted the court's narrow criteria of relevance. The mediators whom we observed generally paid scant regard to the personal circumstances of offenders, many of whom led sad, impoverished lives. The offence in question was often just one further trouble, perhaps a relatively minor one, in a life marked by disrupted family relationships, personality problems, and inadequate skills (including those skills which might secure employment). An acknowledgement of these difficulties was often implicit in the mediators' concern that the offender not be dealt with too severely, but it seldom formed part of the substance of the discussion – in other words, there was little attempt to place the offence in the context of the victim's and the offender's personal circumstances. This meant that the proper apportionment of responsibility was not a matter for discussion – it was assumed to have already been determined by the police or CPS definition of the offence. The question of how, if at all, to make amends was likewise approached with a very blinkered vision. This was disappointing because reparation schemes, one might have thought, would have been well placed to explore precisely those issues – questions of fairness, obligation, degrees of blameworthiness – which courts, handicapped by their formal structures and alien language, cannot address.

This, incidentally, was damaging from the point of view of the *dramatic content* of the mediation sessions which we observed. Anyone who has attended criminal trials will know that courts suck all the drama out of what are, in real life, stupendously dramatic events. True, they offer a limited form of drama in the stylised conflict of professional gladiators – and indeed this forms the substance of many films and television series – but as a reflection of the dramatic impact of tragic events, and of the emotional reaction to those events, courts are quite hopeless, and deliberately so (Christie 1982). Unfortunately, many of the mediation sessions which we observed also lacked drama. This was for one of two reasons: either the events which gave rise to the criminal charge were genuinely trivial; or *the events* were serious, but their treatment in the mediation session lacked psychological reality – usually because the participants were asked to follow a script.

FUTURE DIRECTIONS

The attempt to promote reparation in England and Wales suffered from a lack of coherence, but one has to acknowledge that these would-be mediators faced immense difficulties in any event. The criminal justice system is a mesh of competing interest groups, none of which chose to pay more than lip service to this new concept. There was certainly no endorsement from within the legal profession and even academic interest was muted. There was a new organis-ation, FIRM, but FIRM was unable to attract the political support enjoyed by, for example, the National Association of Victim Support Schemes. There were plenty of potential mediators, but that was another dimension of the problem: reparation schemes would want money in order to expand their operations – and why give money to services which declined to contribute to an already established crimi-nal justice agenda? If reparation was unnecessary for the purposes of diversion; was not applied in serious cases; did not offer an alter-native to custody; did not achieve restitution; did not claim to reduce recidivism . . . what did it have going for it?

A similarly pessimistic view might be arrived at on the basis of experience in other countries. For example, Galaway's research in New Zealand has revealed limited use of that country's reparation provisions (Galaway 1991). He found that reparation featured in only 6.3 per cent of sentences passed in the New Zealand courts and was rarely used as a sole solution. There were also doubts about compli-ance with reparation orders. Galaway concluded that the reparation provision was ineffective in its principal objectives of promoting offender accountability and victim participation. Similarly, Wandrey reports many problems of implementation and a low level of activity in German schemes. These have 'apparently not been successful in convincing the judiciary to promote the programs' development on a practical level' (Wandrey 1991).

The research evidence, then, might incline one to take a pessimistic view of the prospects for reparative justice in the longer term. But before reaching this conclusion it is important to be clear about what these various initiatives were intended to achieve. This is because it is almost inevitable that confused purposes, such as bedevilled the reparation movement in England and Wales, will lead to a sense of frustration and failure. There are, I would suggest, three questions which might help to clarify the position somewhat. They are as follows.

Question One

Should reparation be promoted within *new* programmes, specifically designed for the purpose, or should it be integral to the practice of the existing social control agencies so that it is routinely ordered by courts and supervised by probation officers? In fact there is a range of options, from complete independence on the one hand to total integration (or absorption) on the other. A middle position would be for reparation schemes to seek to *influence* the court, as many do at present, or for reparation to be promoted by probation officers as one element in their therapeutic work with offenders. Each of these positions is tenable, and perhaps it is controversial to assert, as I am inclined to do, that to seek complete independence of the court system would be to consign reparation to a very minor role. Nevertheless, it is important to determine the intended relationship between retributivism, reparation, and 'welfare' approaches – and then to develop institutional arrangements which reflect the agreed policy objectives.

The other two questions follow from this first question.

Question Two

Is it acceptable for reparation to be coerced, as a matter of victim right and offender obligation, or should we cling to the principle of offender autonomy, as use of the term 'mediation' would seem to imply? I have noted that some elements in complete reparation cannot be coerced and succeed; other elements, such as the return of stolen property, can be performed satisfactorily under the inducement of a sentencing discount or as fulfilling the terms of a court order. But it is obviously necessary to decide what degree of importance, if any, one attaches to the principle of voluntariness. We found, in England and Wales, that virtually all reparation schemes *claimed* to adhere to this principle, but that in practice they relied heavily upon the threat of a pending prosecution or court appearance. Offenders and victims alike recognised the ambiguity in this; they understood that it compromised the restoration of trust which reparation performed *without* inducement might have achieved; and they doubted the value of apology delivered in the absence of material reparation and in circumstances where the offender was likely to derive benefit thereby. Reparation which is not coerced may have special value; mandatory material reparation may also, at times, be necessary and desirable; but non-material reparation delivered in the shadow of a pending court appearance will generally fail to convince.

Question Three

Do we regard reparation as a vehicle for achieving decriminalisation, or as a principle of such overriding importance that it should be applied across the whole range of criminal offences, whenever examination of the victim's and offender's circumstances suggests it to be feasible? To employ reparation in the service of diversion is a defensible position, always assuming that diversion is one's principal objective, but it does nothing to challenge the core values of the justice system. It is obviously much more difficult to follow the second course, under which reparative principles (and victim rights) would be enshrined within the justice process, thus, in effect, undermining the criminal/civil dichotomy. This is difficult to contemplate under a procedure which calls for representation of the state and the offender, but not the victim (Campbell 1984). Just as one could not contemplate civil proceedings in the absence of the claimant, so 'reparation' in the absence of the victim is likely to remain peripheral to the main business of the court.

It is for this reason that I feel bound to disagree with Joanna Shapland who has suggested that 'a victim-orientated system . . . would not show many major structural differences from the criminal justice system of today' (Shapland et al, 1985, p. 180). One can illustrate the point by reference to the Criminal Justice Act 1986 which required courts to consider in every relevant case whether a compensation order should be made. It was asserted in the Home Office Green Paper, *Punishment, Custody and the Community*, that this 'would place the responsibility where it belongs by requiring offenders to pay for the injury, loss or damage they have caused' (Home Office 1988, para. 2.8). There is one thing wrong with this – one thing missing. It is impossible to imagine magistrates or judges giving priority to compensation, or to any other form of reparation, unless the victim is present in court – and not only present, but heard. The test of whether the Home Office is serious about compensation in the context of criminal proceedings lies in the provision which it is prepared to make to ensure that victims are invited to attend court, offered representation, and permitted to influence the conduct and outcome of the proceedings. This suggestion may seem far-fetched, but it is what is required if we are to have a justice system based on reparative principles.

There is of course an objection of principle, or one might say of justice theory, to this proposal in that it is commonly asserted that crime is an injury to the state rather than to the individual. In 1985 Enoch Powell made a speech to the Cambridge University Conservative Association on just this theme. Unfortunately, Powell, in common with other advocates of the status quo, failed to deal with the implicit challenge of reparation to the present practice of hiving off certain kinds of harmful behaviour and calling them 'crime', whilst allowing much other harmful behaviour to be regarded as a civil wrong, or no wrong at all as far as our courts are concerned. What is so sacrosanct about the present boundaries of crime? Powell seemed to presume that the present division between harms which are classed as criminal offences and harms which are classed as civil wrongs is beyond question. But that line, and its implications for control of outcome by victim and offender (or 'the disputants'), might be re-drawn.

The question of what kinds of harm should be dealt with as criminal offences is a difficult one and relates to our concept of citizenship. Sovereign authority does not penetrate every nook and cranny of our lives. We allow it to govern some relatively minor matters (parking on double yellow lines) but not major ones (honouring father and mother; abandoning spouse; failure to maintain children). Perhaps Powell was too self-confident in proclaiming what is due to the sovereign authority. He declared himself opposed to 'the fragmentation of the life of society into an infinite number of autonomous relationships and inter-actions between the individuals composing it', but this is not to challenge the making of reparation for those acts which are currently classified as criminal offences. The essential difference between crime and civil wrong (leaving aside the different penalties that may result) is that in the latter case reparation must be pursued by the individual complainant. In both instances the rights infringed may be shared by more people than are harmed on the one occasion; it is simply that under the former definition the state prosecutes.

It is impossible to determine which acts fall 'naturally' within the scope of the criminal law. At the margins, where the reparation schemes which we studied tended to locate themselves, there is evident scope for de-criminalising some actions which give rise to a criminal charge. And of course there are a great many *potentially* criminal acts which are, in practice, dealt with in the private realm. Many assaults, for example, are handled in this way. Some victims will define a given behaviour as criminal while others will regard it as a purely private matter. Furthermore, social attitudes and criminal definitions may change, as witness the recent criminalisation of that form of financial misbehaviour known as 'insider dealing', or the acceptance that rape may be perpetrated within marriage. Christie observes that within some societies a great many acts are regarded as criminal, whereas in others the social arrangements are such that those same acts are perceived as expressions of conflicting interests (Christie 1982, p. 11). At the same time it is important to acknowledge that many crimes *cannot* plausibly be re-classified in this way. This applies in relation even to quite minor matters – for example (to take a couple of cases outlined in earlier chapters), to occasional shoplifting from a large store, or to hoax 999 calls. Blagg and his colleagues, in their research on the South Yorkshire reparation scheme, noted a preponderance of commercial victims. This in turn meant that there were limited opportunities for negotiation (Smith et al, 1989). One reason for this may be that the kind of problem which we are likely to define as 'a quarrel' or 'a dispute' is likely to involve a prior personal relationship and it is precisely within this kind of relationship that the injured party is likely to react by avoidance or by 'lumping' the offending behaviour (Felstiner 1974).

These are matters which need to be further explored. For the moment I would prefer to be cautious about endorsing the Christie thesis that reparative principles should be placed at the heart of criminal justice. This is because we do not know *how much* or *what kinds* of reparations are feasible across the range of circumstances which currently give rise to a criminal prosecution. Research on victim/offender reparation schemes is of minimal assistance here. What is required is a study of the potential for a reparative component across a range of cases currently prosecuted through our criminal courts, with none of the confusion attendant upon the selection of cases being based partly upon their being low tariff, or upon their having some other potential for diversion or mitigation. At the moment it tends to be assumed that most offenders have little to offer victims by way of explanation or reassurance and, secondly, that adequate material compensation can only be provided by the state. But this is something one might wish to test. Equality of treatment as between persons who commit similar offences does not mean that all should have the *same* treatment. It would be necessary to look closely at a range of offences, and at the social circumstances of the perpetrators and their victims, in order to determine what forms of reparation, if any, were (a) feasible; and (b) just.

But there is another consideration which is fundamental to any discussion of the scope for mediation (as a process) and reparation (as an outcome) in response to criminal acts. There are occasions, perhaps in relation to more serious offences, where the scope for reparation is so limited that it would not justify the court's abandoning an appropriate level of retribution in order to permit some vestigial element of reparation to be performed. This objection, I would suggest, forms the basis of a certain intuitive resistance to the reparation case and it needs to be addressed. It has a reputable philosophical underpinning in the argument that criminal proceedings have a moral purpose which civil actions, geared to achieving compensation, do not possess (MacCormick 1978). Civil law coerces a moral duty – the duty to make reparation if one causes harm. Criminal proceedings may have this as one end product, but their principal function is to express social disapprobation. The retributive paradigm focuses upon the violation of social norms; in other words, it has *symbolic* significance (Hay 1975, p. 58; Bussman 1991). It need not be effective, according to any of the traditional utilitarian measures, in order for this symbolic purpose to be fulfilled.

If we view the criminal law in terms of its capacity to promote deference and maintain order, which is what Hay and Bussman argue, then a system built on an attempt to individualise and particularise justice – however reasonable it might be in specific cases – would not be an adequate substitute because it would lack symbolic power. Mediation, being geared to private resolution, cannot replicate the symbolism of the retributive paradigm. Having a private character, it cannot symbolise our essential social values – which means that it cannot replace the public performance of the criminal process. This strikes me as a persuasive argument and I am grateful to Kai Bussman for a preliminary view of the paper in which he develops his thesis. There are however a number of caveats which one might wish to enter.

First, the public performance of *punishment* (as distinct from the determination of guilt) has already all but disappeared, and yet Western society seems to manage without the opportunity for norm clarification afforded by public whippings and hangings, displaying offenders in the stocks, and so on. Perhaps the criminal trial (as reported in the press and on television) fulfils this function for us. The second caveat is more fundamental in that it goes to the heart of what we mean by reparative justice. Bussman assumes that reparation is necessarily to be determined through mediation – that is to say, in private. But this is a big assumption. One can imagine major transgressions (and, from the victim's point of view, major tragedies) being discussed *publicly* and yet in terms of a reparative paradigm. The recent Guinness share-dealing scandal in the UK was dealt with partly along these lines, although a retributive element was imposed in addition to the compensation ordered. Arguments about blame and responsibility, and about compensation, do not necessarily lack symbolic power – or, indeed, dramatic content. Big libel trials, of which we have had a spate in the UK of late, offer a further illustration of this. Nils Christie, indeed, argues the case for lay courts and a reparative model precisely on the basis that these would afford greater opportunity for norm-clarification (Christie 1977). The conclusion of this argument must depend on how one thinks social values are best transmitted – whether through professionally dominated set-piece denunciations of the most wicked human conduct, or by means of lay participation, informal procedures, and a reparative paradigm.

Perhaps the answer is that we need both. This, indeed, is Bussman's conclusion. He suggests a model of 'reflexive law' (derived from Teubner 1983) under which mediation schemes would handle cases autonomously, with the criminal law providing rules governing the referral of cases to what would in effect be an autonomous sub-system; the public prosecutor would retain responsibility for dealing with selected, severe cases, enabling the criminal law to fulfil its symbolic function. As Bussman observes, there need not be very many such cases in order for this symbolic purpose to be fulfilled. This proposal will no doubt strike some readers as fanciful, but one could equally regard it as an eminently practical measure, enabling our over-burdened criminal courts to concentrate upon the only tasks which they are fitted to perform, namely, the determination of guilt or innocence and, secondly, the public denunciation of a relatively few grossly anti-social acts.

The problem about this proposal (aside from the professional opposition which it would of course arouse) is that we do not, as yet, have an effective reparation practice upon which to base such a model. At least, we do not have one in England and Wales. So whilst I might wish to conclude these reflections on an up-beat note, I am conscious of the limited progress made to date. The reparation schemes which we observed sought to appease a punishing system whose destructive potential they well understood. They paid little heed to the needs of victims and their approach to mediation reflected a particular response to conflict and threat – a deflecting, anxious response which conveyed the message that they wished only that other people approached these matters more as they did. Their deliberate focus upon the trivial was in keeping with the supplicatory position in which they were placed, or placed themselves. It reflected what they took to be the weakness of their position. But there is evidence in this book to suggest that, freed from the obligation to appease a punishing system, reparation schemes can do something which criminal courts cannot hope to do, namely, tackle perennially important questions of responsibility and justification, thus enabling them to 'do justice' in ways not open to a judge operating under legal rules (Silbey 1981). If professional prejudice can be set aside, they may, in this way, demonstrate their capacity to respond effectively to serious harm.

Bibliography

All-Party Penal Affairs Group (1984) *A New Deal for Victims*, NACRO: London.

Atkinson, J.M. and Drew, P. (1979) *Order in Court*, Humanities Press: London.

Auerbach, J.S. (1983) *Justice without Law?*, Clarendon Press: Oxford.

Baldwin, J. and McConville, M. (1977) *Negotiated Justice*, Martin Robertson: Oxford.

Balint, M. (1951) *On Punishment*, Unpublished paper.

Barnett, R.E. (1977) 'Restitution: A New Paradigm of Criminal Justice', 80/87 *Ethics*, 279–301.

Bayfield, T. (1989) 'A fantasy cloaked in false saintliness', *The Independent*, 3.6.89, p. 16.

Becker, H. (1963) *Outsiders: Studies in the Sociology of Deviance*, Free Press: New York.

Blackstone, W. (1778) *Commentaries on the Laws of England*, Clarendon Press: Oxford.

Blagg, H. (1985) 'Reparation and Justice for Juveniles: the Corby Experience', *British Journal of Criminology*, Vol. 25, 267–279.

Blagg, H. (1986) 'Review of Punishment and Restitution by C.F. Abel and F.H. Marsh', Greenwood Press, *British Journal of Criminology*, Vol. 26, 303–306.

Blumberg, A.S. (1967) 'The Practice of Law as a Confidence Game: Organizational Co-option of a Profession', *Law and Society Review*, Vol. 1, 15–39.

Bottoms, A.E. and McClean, J.D. (1976) *Defendants in the Criminal Process*, Routledge and Kegan Paul: London.

Braithwaite, J. (1989) *Crime, Shame and Reintegration*, Cambridge University Press: Cambridge.

Brittan, L. (1984) Home Secretary's Speech to the Holborn Law Society, 14.3.84.

Bussman, K. (1991) 'Morality, Symbolism and Criminal Law: Chances and Limits of Mediation Programs', *ARW Workshop*, Il Ciocco, Italy, April 8–12.

Cain, M. (1988) 'Beyond Informal Justice', in *Informal Justice?* (Matthews, R., ed.), Sage: London.

Campbell, T. (1984) 'Compensation as Punishment', *University of New South Wales Law Journal*, Vol. 7, 338–361.

Chadwick, O. (1975) *The Secularization of the European Mind in the Nineteenth Century*, Cambridge University Press: Cambridge.

Chinkin, C.M. and Griffiths, R.C. (1980) 'Resolving Conflict by Mediation', *New Law Journal*, pp. 6–8.

Christie, N. (1977) 'Conflicts as Property', *British Journal of Criminology*, Vol. 17/1.

Christie, N. (1982) *Limits to Pain*, Martin Robertson: Oxford.

Christie, N. (1986) 'Crime Control as Drama', *Journal of Law and Society*, Vol. 13/1.

Coates, R.B. and Gehm, J. (1989) 'An Empirical Assessment', in *Mediation and Criminal Justice* (Wright, M. and Galaway, B., eds), Sage: London.

Cohen, S. (1985) *Visions of Social Control*, Polity Press: Oxford.

Davis, G. (1988) *Partisans and Mediators*, Clarendon Press: Oxford.

Davis, G., Boucherat, J. and Watson, D. (1987) 'A Preliminary Study of Victim/Offender Mediation and Reparation Schemes in England and Wales', *Research and Planning Unit Paper 42*, The Home Office: London.

Davis, G., Boucherat, J. and Watson, D. (1988) 'Reparation in the service of diversion: the subordination of a good idea', *The Howard Journal*, Vol. 27/2.

Davis, G., Boucherat, J. and Watson, D. (1989) 'Pre-court decision-making in juvenile justice', *British Journal of Criminology*, Vol. 29/3.

Davis, G. and Roberts, M. (1988) *Access to Agreement*, Open University Press: Milton Keynes.

Davis, R. (1980) *Mediation and Arbitration as Alternative to Prosecution in Felony Arrest Cases: An Evaluation of the Brooklyn Dispute Resolution Center*, VERA Institute of Justice: New York.

Dünkell, F. and Rössner, D. (1989) 'Law and Practice of Victim/Offender Agreements', in *Mediation and Criminal Justice* (Wright, M. and Galaway, G., eds), Sage: London.

Dunpark, Lord (1977) *Reparation by the Offender to the Victim in Scotland* (Dunpark Report), Cmnd. 6802, HMSO: Edinburgh.

Felstiner, W. (1974) 'Influences of Social Organisation on Dispute Processing', *Law and Society Review*, Vol. 9(1): 63–94.

FIRM (1986) *An Interim Response to 'Reparation: A Discussion Document'*, Forum for Initiatives in Reparation and Mediation, 19 London End, Beaconsfield, Bucks HP9 2HN.

FIRM (1988) 'Repairing the Damage', *Proceedings of the First National Symposium on Mediation and Criminal Justice*, Forum for Initiatives in Reparation and Mediation, 19 London End, Beaconsfield, Bucks HP9 2HN.

Foucault, M. (1975) *Discipline and Punish*, Penguin: Harmondsworth.

Frehsee, D. (1987) Schadenswiedergutmachung als Instrument strafrechtlicher Sozialkontrolle, Berlin.

Galaway, B. (1991) 'Challenges to Implementation of Reparation as a Restorative Sanction: The New Zealand Experience', *ARW Workshop*, Il Ciocco, Italy, April 8–12.

Garland, D. (1990) *Punishment and Modern Society*, Clarendon Press: Oxford.

Garton, A. (1986) *Preliminary Report on The Leeds Reparation Scheme*, Unpublished Research Paper.

Gehm, J. (1990) 'Mediated Victim–Offender Restitution Agreements: An Exploratory Analysis of Factors Related to Victim Participation', in *Crimi-*

nal Justice, Restitution and Reconciliation, (Galaway, B., and Hudson, J., eds), Criminal Justice Press: Monsey, New York.

Giller, H. (1986) 'Is there a role for a juvenile court?' *The Howard Journal*, Vol. 25/3, pp. 161–71.

Grümer, H. (1984) 'Kommunikation in Arbeitsgerichtsverhandlungen – Versuch einer Analyse', in *Rechtssoziologische Studien zur Arbeitsgerichtsbarkeit*, (Rottleuthner, H., ed.), Nomos: Baden-Baden.

Guedalia, L.J. (1979) Predicting Recidivism of Juvenile Delinquents on Restitutionary Probation from Selected Background, Subject and Program Variables: Unpublished doctoral dissertation, American University: Washington, DC.

Haley, J.O. (1989) 'Confession, Repentance and Absolution', in *Mediation and Criminal Justice* (Wright, M. and Galaway, B., eds), Sage: London.

Hampton, J. (1984) 'The Moral Education Theory of Punishment', *Philosophy and Public Affairs*, Vol. 13/3.

Harding, J. (1982) *Victims and Offenders: Needs and Responsibilities*, Bedford Square Press: London.

Harding, J. (1989) 'Reconciling Mediation with Criminal Justice', in *Mediation and Criminal Justice* (Wright, M. and Galaway, B., eds), Sage: London.

Hartmann, A. (1989) Begleitforschung für die Modellprojekte in München und Landshut, in *Täter-Opfer-Ausgleich*, (Marks, E., and Rössner, D., eds), Forum: Bonn.

Hay, D. (1975) 'Property, Authority and the Criminal Law', in *Albion's Fatal Tree*, (Hay, D. et al), Penguin: Harmondsworth.

Hay, D., Linebaugh, P., Winslow, C., Rule, J.G. and Thompson, E.P. (1975) *Albion's Fatal Tree*, Allen Lane: London. (Reprinted 1988 by Penguin Books.)

Hofrichter, R. (1980) 'Techniques of Victim Involvement in Restitution', in *Victims, Offenders, and Alternative Sanctions* (Hudson, J. and Galaway, B., eds), Lexington Books: Lexington, Mass.

Home Office (1984) *Cautioning by the Police: A Consultative Document*, HMSO: London.

Home Office (1986) *Reparation: A Discussion Document*, Home Office: London.

Home Office (1986a) *Criminal Justice: A Working Paper* (Revised Edition), Home Office: London.

Home Office (1988) *Punishment, Custody and the Community*, Cmnd. 424, HMSO: London.

Home Office (1990) *Crime, Justice and Protecting the Public*, Cmnd. 965, HMSO: London.

Hudson, J. and Galaway, B. (1977) *Restitution in Criminal Justice*, D.C. Heath: Lexington, Mass.

Hughes, S.P. and Schneider, A.L. (1989) Victim–Offender Mediation: A Survey of Program Characteristics and Perceptions of Effectiveness, *Crime and Delinquency*, Vol. 46/2.

Ignatieff, M. (1989) *A Just Measure of Pain*, Penguin: Harmondsworth.

Kuhn, A., Rudolph, M., Wandrey, M., and Will, H-D. (1989) '*Tat-Sachen*' *als Konflikt*, Forum: Bonn.

Launay, G. (1985) 'Bringing Victims and Offenders Together: A Comparison of Two Models', *The Howard Journal*, Vol. 24/3.

Launay, G. (1987) 'Victim–Offender Conciliation' in *Applying Psychology to Imprisonment: Theory and Practice* (McGurk, B., Thornton, D. and Williams, M., eds), HMSO: London.

Lemert, E. (1967) *Human Deviance, Social Problems and Social Control*, Prentice Hall: New Jersey.

Lukes, S. (1973) *Individualism*, Basil Blackwell: Oxford.

MacCormick, D.N. (1978) 'The Obligation of Reparation', *Proceedings of the Aristotelian Society*, Vol. 78: 175–193.

Maguire, M. and Corbett, C. (1987) *The Effects of Crime and the Work of Victims Support Schemes*, Gower: London.

Maguire, M. and Pointing, J. (1988) *Victims of Crime: A New Deal?* Open University Press: Milton Keynes.

Maine, Sir Henry (1861) *Ancient Law*, Murray: London.

Marshall, T.F. (1985) *Alternatives to Criminal Courts*, Gower: Aldershot.

Marshall, T.F. (1986) '*Monitoring of Mediation and Reparation Schemes: Early Indications from Data Available*', June 1986, Home Office: London.

Marshall, T.F. (1988) 'Informal Justice: The British Experience', in *Informal Justice?* (Matthews, R., ed.), Sage: London.

Marshall, T.F. and Merry, S. (1990) *Crime and Accountability: Victim/Offender Mediation in Practice*, HMSO: London.

Marshall, T. and Walpole, M. (1985) 'Bringing People Together: Mediation and Reparation Projects in Great Britain', *Research and Planning Unit Paper 33*, Home Office: London.

Mawby, R. and Gill, M. (1987) *Crime Victims*, Tavistock: London.

McAnany, P. D. (1978) 'Restitution as Idea and Practice: The Retributive Prospect', in *Offender Restitution in Theory and Action* (Hudson, J. and Galaway, B., eds), Lexington Books: Lexington, Mass.

Merry, S.E. (1989) 'Myth and Practice in the Mediation Process', in *Mediation and Criminal Justice* (Wright, M. and Galaway, B., eds), Sage: London.

Messmer, H. (1989) 'Tackling the Conflict', in *The State as Parent*, (Galaway, B. and Hudson, J., eds), Kluwer: The Netherlands.

Messmer, H. (1991) 'The Effectiveness of Victim–Offender Mediation', *ARW Workshop*, Il Ciocco, Italy, April 8–12.

Mika, H. (1991) 'Mediation Interventions and Restorative Justice: Responding to the Astructural Bias', *ARW Workshop*, Il Ciocco, Italy, April 8–12.

Moberly, E. (1978) *Suffering, Innocent and Guilty*, SPCK: London.

Moberly, W. (1968) *The Ethics of Punishment*, Faber & Faber: London.

National Association of Probation Officers (NAPO) (1985) *Policy Document on Reparation*, 314 Chivalry Road, London SW11 1HT.

Nelken, D. (1986) 'Reparation Seminar', *Mediation*, Vol. 3/1.

O'Brien, E. (1986) *Asking the Victim: A Study of the Attitudes of Some Victims of Crime to Reparation and the Criminal Justice System*, Gloucestershire Probation Service.

Peachey, D.E. (1989) 'The Kitchener Experiment', in *Mediation and Criminal Justice*, (Wright, M. and Galaway B., eds), Sage: London.

Powell, J.E. (1985) *Speech to the Cambridge University Conservative Association*, 20.10.85, *The Times*, 21.10.85.

Pratt, J. (1986) 'Diversion from the Juvenile Court', *British Journal of Criminology*, Vol. 26, 212.

Priestley, P. (1977) 'Victims: The Key to Reform', *Christian Action Journal*, Summer, pp. 12–13.

Priestley, P. and McGuire, J. (1985) *Offending Behaviour: Skills and Stratagems for Going Straight*, Batsford Academic and Educational: London.

Radzinowicz, L. (1948) *A History of English Criminal Law and its Administration from 1750–1948* – Part 1, p. 77, Stevens: London.

Reeves, H. (1984) 'The Victim and Reparation', *Probation Journal*, Vol. 31/4.

Reeves, H. (1989) 'The Victim Support Perspective', in *Mediation and Criminal Justice* (Wright, M. and Galaway B., eds), Sage: London.

Roberts, S. (1979) *Order and Dispute*, Penguin: Harmondsworth.

Roberts, S. (1983) 'Mediation in Family Disputes', *Modern Law Review*, Vol. 46/5.

Rock, P. (1986) *A View from the Shadows*, Clarendon Press: Oxford.

Rock, P. (1990) *Helping Victims of Crime*, Clarendon Press: Oxford.

Ryle, G. (1963) *The Concept of Mind*, Penguin: Harmondsworth.

Schafer, S. (1960) *Compensation and Restitution to Victims of Crime*, Patterson Smith Publishing Corp: Montclair, NJ; Stevens: London.

Schmitz, C. (1988) 'Die Braunschweiger Projektpraxis in Zahlen', *Braunschweiger Hefte zum Jugend, Sozial/ und Gesundheitswesen*, Vol. 12, 125–142.

Schneider, A.L. (1986) 'Restitution and Recidivism Rates of Juvenile Offenders: Results from Four Experimental Studies', *Criminology*, Vol. 24/3.

Schreckling, J. (1990) *Täter-Opfer-Ausgleich nach Jugenstraftaten in Köln*, Bundesministerium der Justiz: Bonn.

Schur, E. (1973) *Radical Non-Intervention: Rethinking the Delinquency Problem*, Prentice Hall: New Jersey.

Shapland, J. (1984) 'Victims, the Criminal Justice System and Compensation', *British Journal of Criminology*, Vol. 24, 131–149.

Shapland, J., Wilmore, J. and Duff, P. (1985) *Victims in the Criminal Justice System*, Gower: Aldershot.

Shikita, M. (1982) 'Integrated approach to effective administration of criminal and juvenile justice', in *Criminal Justice in Asia: The Quest for an Integrated Approach*, UNAFEI: Tokyo.

Silbey, S. (1981) 'Making Sense of the Lower Courts', *The Justice System Journal*, Vol. 6, 13–27.

Smith, D., Blagg, H., and Derricourt, N. (1985) *Victim–Offender Mediation Project: Report to Chief Officers' Group*, South Yorkshire Probation Service.

Smith, D., Blagg, H., and Derricourt, N. (1989) 'Mediation in the Shadow of the Law: The South Yorkshire Experience', in *Informal Justice?* (Matthews, R., ed.), Sage: London.

Sykes, G.M. and Matza, D. (1957) 'Techniques of Neutralisation: A Theory of Delinquency', *American Sociological Review*, Vol. 22, 664–670.

Teubner, G. (1983) 'Substantive and Reflexive Elements in Modern Law', *Law and Society Review*, Vol. 17/2, 239–285.

Thatcher, A. (1991) *The Religious Roots of Mediation and Reparation*, Unpublished research paper.

Thomas, P. (1986) *The Aims and Outcomes of Social Policy Research*, Croom Helm: London.

Thompson, E.P. (1975) *Whigs and Hunters*, Allen Lane: London.

Tomasic, R. (1982) 'Mediation as an Alternative to Adjudication: Rhetoric and Reality in the Neighbourhood Justice Movement', in *Neighbourhood Justice: An Assessment of an Emerging Idea* (Tomasic, R. and Feeley, M., eds), Longman: New York.

Umbreit, M.S. (1985) *Crime and Reconciliation: Creative Options for Victims and Offenders*, Abingdon Press: Nashville.

Umbreit, M.S. (1985a) *Victim Offender Mediation: Conflict Resolution and Restitution*, US Department of Justice: Washington D.C.

Umbreit, M.S. (1986) 'Victim Offender Mediation and Judicial Leadership', *Judicature*, December.

Umbreit, M.S. (1988) 'Mediation of Victim Offender Conflict', *Journal of Dispute Resolution*, University of Missouri School of Law, Columbia.

Umbreit, M.S. (1989) 'Victims Seeking Fairness, Not Revenge: Toward Restorative Justice', *Federal Probation*, September.

Umbreit, M.S. (1990) 'The Meaning of Fairness to Burglary Victims', in *Criminal Justice, Restitution and Reconciliation*, (Galaway, B., and Hudson, J., eds), Criminal Justice Press: Monsey, NY.

Umbreit, M.S. (1991) 'An Evaluation of the Center for Victim Offender Mediation in Minneapolis', *Journal of the International Association of Residential and Community Alternatives*, IARCA: LaCrosse, WI.

Vennard, J. (1976) 'Justice and Recompense for Victims of Crime', *New Society*, Vol. 35, 378–380.

Wagatsuma, H. and Rosett, A. (1986) 'The Implications of Apology: Law and Culture in Japan and the United States', *Law and Society Review*, Vol. 20, 461–498.

Walgrave, L. (1991) 'Mediation and Community Service: Why should it be better?' *ARW Workshop*, Il Ciocco, Italy, April 8–12.

Walklate, S. (1989) *Victimology: the Victim and the Criminal Justice Process*, Unwin Hyman: London.

Walster, E., Berscheid, E. and Walster, G.W. (1973) 'New Directions in Equity Research', *Journal of Personality and Social Psychology*, Vol. 25, 151–176.

Wandrey, M. (1991) 'Organized Demands on Mediation Programs: Problems of Realization', *ARW Workshop*, Il Ciocco, Italy, April 8–12.

Wasik, M. (1978) 'The Place of Compensation in the Penal System', *Criminal Law Review*, 599.

Watson, D., Boucherat, J. and Davis, G. (1989) 'Reparation for Retributivists', in *Mediation and Criminal Justice* (Wright, M. and Galaway, B., eds), Sage: London.

Wright, M. (1981) 'Crime and reparation: breaking the penal logjam', *New Society*, 444–446.

Wright, M. (1982) *Making Good*, Burnett Books: London.

Young, R. (1987) *Research Report on the Wolverhampton Reparation Scheme*, Institute of Judicial Administration: University of Birmingham.

Young, R. (1987a) Research Report on the Coventry Reparation Scheme, Institute of Judicial Administration: University of Birmingham.

Young, R. (1989) 'Reparation as Mitigation', in *Criminal Law Review*, 463–472.

Zehr, H. (1985) *Retributive Justice, Restorative Justice*, Elkhart, Indiana, MCC U.S. Office of Criminal Justice Occasional Paper.

Zehr, H. (1986) 'Howard Zehr on British Mediation', *Mediation*, Winter, Vol. 2/2.

Zehr, H. (1988) 'Reparation: Where from Here?', in 'Repairing the Damage', *Proceedings of the First National Symposium on Mediation and Criminal Justice*, FIRM: Beaconsfield.

Zehr, H. (1990) *Changing Lenses*, Herald Press: Scottdale, PA.

Zehr, H., and Umbreit, M.S. (1982) Victim Offender Reconciliation: An Incarceration Substitute? *Federal Probation*, Vol. 46/4.

Index